Get Well, Be Well, Stay Well

Get Well, Be Well, Stay Well
with herbal plants

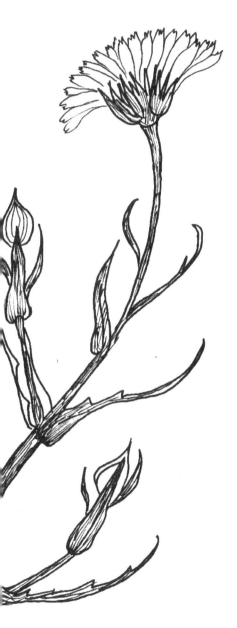

written & illustrated by
Lise M. Fuller

Cover illustrations by Lise M. Fuller
Edited by Aubrey Restifo
Book design by The Troy Book Makers

Printed in the United States of America

The Troy Book Makers • Troy, New York • thetroybookmakers.com

To order additional copies of this title, contact your favorite local bookstore or visit www.shoptbmbooks.com

ISBN: 978-1-61468-473-2

MEDICAL DISCLAIMER

The following information is intended for general information purposes only. Individuals should always see their health care providers before administering any suggestions made in this book. Any application of the material set forth in the following pages is at the reader's discretion and is his or her sole responsibility.

ACKNOWLEDGMENTS

*To all the people who never wavered in their
belief in the healing powers of plants.*

TABLE OF CONTENTS

SECTION 2 • *How to Get Well*

SECTION 3 • *Be Well, Stay Well*

SECTION 4 • *Information*

PROLOGUE

How do you know what you know about herbs?

As I sat down to write the "About the Author" section I decided not to list all of my life accomplishments and particulars, but rather use the opportunity to answer a question which I have been asked time and time again. My experience in learning, teaching and helping people use herbal plants reflects the type of society we live in, and its attitudes towards what kind of medicine is acceptable and legal.

I have always loved plants and being outside. I grew up in the suburban world of the 1950s and 60s. Cutting the grass was as close as I'd get to working with plants. I created my first vegetable garden in my twenties and have been gardening ever since.

If I had stuck to gardening vegetables and flowers, my life would have been simple and uncomplicated; instead, I became interested in using plants for medicine. The concept seemed simple enough. I was growing plants for food which nurtured the body, so why wouldn't the plants also work to help treat the various health issues that people faced all the time? That was the way it was done throughout history. All the other countries used botanical medicine. What was the big deal? It turned out that using plants for medicines would be a very big deal in this country.

In the 1960s and 70s, there was a huge "back to the land" movement. I lived in the hills of the Berkshires where I grew a huge vegetable garden. Among the vegetables I grew were culinary herbs. I had an immense amount of parsley one year so I started to look into how to preserve plants which led me to dry the parsley in a homemade solar dyer. I was amazed by the dehydrated parsley: it smelled fresh and sweet and was bright green and full of vitality—unlike anything I'd ever bought in a grocery or health food store.

Back then people were doing exactly what I was doing: growing all kinds of plants and herbs, making herbal plant preparations, reading about how to use herbs in old books and sharing their knowledge with each other. There was an herbal renaissance or herb revival of sorts in those years. People were interested in all sorts of alternative methods such as gardening organically and living "off the grid" (as we called it then). I remember poring over my issues of organic gardening and seeing new ideas about just about everything. We were going to reinvent the world.

I attended one of the first alternative energy fairs held at the University of Massachusetts in the early seventies. I bought plans for a solar dehydrator to dry my herbs from my huge garden. There were so many innovative ideas about using alternative energy. It was an exciting time for different ideas to flourish and take hold.

When I moved back north after living all over the U.S., I revisited my interest in medicinal plants and decided to get serious about studying plants that worked as medicine.

Education of an Herbalist

My first herbal workshop took place in Vermont. We went out into the teacher's garden. I remember thinking, "What an unkempt, weedy garden!" We proceeded to pick the weeds instead of the plants, brought them back to the kitchen, and cooked them up and ate them. It was a revelation. I was raised to be afraid of "weeds": they were to be eradicated from lawns at all costs. It turns out that most weeds are edible, filled with vitamins and minerals, and are perhaps even better for you than most vegetables. Who knew? We dug burdock roots which seemed to go down to the core of the earth and picked nettles without gloves. I also learned to dowse for water from a guy in his mid-80s. That was all in one afternoon. I was hooked.

Twenty-five years ago I attended one of the first Northeast Women's Herbal Conferences. (This conference is still held today: www.womensherbalconference.com.) I was struck by the camaraderie of those courageous women and the confidence with which they pursued their interest in medicinal plants regardless of what society deemed acceptable. I was exposed to so many new ideas about plants, food, healing and even plant crafts. The herbal world seem to include a little bit of everything. I remember how much fun it was to make herbal elixirs or liquors. Adele Dawson, an herbalist from Vermont, dumped what looked like a five pound bag of white sugar, a bottle of vodka and a lot of strange herbal plants into a gallon-size deli pickle glass jar. She told us to let it steep for several weeks and then you'd have it: a delicious liquor.

Back then, the way to learn about using herbal plants was to learn directly from the people who were using them. You learned by spending considerable amounts of time with knowledgeable herbalists in their homes, gardens, and favorite wild places to learn firsthand how they grew and used plants. These people "walked their talk" and held workshops, apprenticeship programs and conferences all over the country. I attended many workshops throughout the northeast and Canada. We had wonderful herbal gatherings where plant loving people set up tables, shared their knowledge and sold their latest herbal wares. These herbalists opened up their hearts and homes to others who had the desire to learn about herbal plants. I think now about how different such a thing is from the behavior of our sanctioned health care professionals, who only have fifteen minutes to spend with people. I can't imagine those professionals opening up their homes to share their knowledge in the same way.

Many herbalists have written books about their experiences with the plants. Seek out books written by people who have firsthand knowledge about using plants as opposed to books which contain scientific "facts" about the plants. You will notice that every herbalist has favorite plants which work for them. This book is filled with my favorite plants and recipes that have worked for me. As you work with plants you will develop your own relationships with certain herbal plants. Having a relationship with plants is our birthright as human beings. It is not necessary to have American Indian blood or to be a certain gender to be able to use and understand the plant kingdom. It is open to everyone.

Fear of Plants

Every plant workshop and gathering I attended always included so much more than just plants. Early on in my pursuit of herbal knowledge I watched a documentary called 'Burning Times', which is part of a trilogy on women's history. It is distributed by Direct Cinema Limited. For the first time, I heard about the history of the persecution of women by the

Catholic Church in Europe during the middle ages. Village women healers were branded "witches" and burned at the stake or tortured to death so
that the church could suppress their healing plant knowledge. As I learned
about this before the internet existed, such information was not widely
known. I was shocked that I had never heard about this part of women's
history, nor the long history of the suppression of plant knowledge. This
part of my herbal education became extremely useful when I tried to make
sense of the fear that I encountered when I started teaching : the fear of
using herbal plants. I was called a "witch" many times (the term intended
to be an insult), but the anger and insults made no sense to me—after all,
it was the nineties not the 1600s. The fear seemed to be directed at much
more than the plants themselves. It seemed that those horrible times were
still embedded in people's psyches, especially in those of the women that I
would teach and see at herbal gatherings.

The role of an herbalist has always existed throughout history, so it is
important to seek out older books and information to see how herbalism
was at one time a common part of our society. I had the privilege to meet
the late Juliette de Bairacli Levy, an herbalist in her 80s who had traveled
all over the world as an herbalist, lived with the gypsies in Europe, and
practiced her art everywhere she went. She was famous for her book, *The
Complete Herbal Handbook for the Farm and Stable*, and for her work with
animals. She wasn't keen on working with people: her love was her dogs,
Afghan wolfhounds, which she bred with great success. To get a feeling
for her life as an herbalist, the documentary "Juliette of the Herbs" by
Tish Streeten gives a picture of a person devoted to the world of medicinal
plants. Although there are many books that discuss herbalists, one of my
favorites is 1886's *The Country of the Pointed Firs* by Sarah Orne Jewett
which depicts a life of an herbalist on the coast of Maine. Perhaps I enjoy
it because I am from Maine and recognize the plants that are mentioned
in the book.

Our country has a rich tradition of using plants: it goes without saying
that the indiginous people of this continent used plants for healing purposes. They taught the settlers their plant knowledge. The immigrant cultures also brought their plants and seeds with them when they came here.
Currently there is a renewed interest in native plants, referring to the plants
that were here before Columbus. The eclectic physicians who practiced
during the late 1800s used plants in their practices. They left a treasure-
trove of their herbal work behind, work that is preserved today at the Lloyd

Library in Cincinnati, Ohio. This country was a botanical wonderland and the book "Native American Ethobotany" by Daniel E. Moerman ilustrates the immense work it took to catalogue the plants from the "new world".

In fact everywhere you look around the world you will find examples of plant-based healing systems. In India, you'll find the Ayurvedic Tradition. In China, you'll find Traditional Chinese Medicine (or TCM as it's called). In Europe and elsewhere, homeopathy became a very popular plant-based system over the turn of the last century. A good book to read to better understand the history of medicinal plant use is Barbara Griggs' *Green Pharmacy*.

The Sciences

Although I knew a lot about plants and the ways in which they worked in the body, I felt that I needed to grasp such phenomena from a scientific perspective as well. I attended my local community college to explore plants as they are taught in this country.

I loved studying the sciences. I was amazed by the creative thinking that was involved in the creation of experiments to test and prove new theories. I thought I met some pretty eccentric people in the herbal world, but after studying botany I found that the scientific world was filled with amazing, eccentric and creative people as well.

I was lucky to study with a botany teacher who believed in the importance of the scientific method and how it applied to our world. Our physicians train as scientists. This explains their comfort with using drugs as opposed to plants. As I learned then, chemical drugs could be measured as opposed to plants which could be difficult to measure with the then-current scientific methods (scientific methods are constantly being updated: my course took place over twenty years ago). At the time, the attitude toward science I'd encounter most in the herbal community was proudly "anti-science". As I studied the sciences, I realized that this attitude signaled that they opposed the limitations of the medical system as it existed at that time. Twenty-five years ago there was no such thing as acupuncture or aromatherapy as a healing system. In New York State they didn't allow chiropractors into the health insurance system. When my friend took her massage therapist exam, they checked her hands to see if she was wearing nail polish (to determine whether or not she was a sex worker!)

The atmosphere of the science building was in direct contrast to that of the outside herbal environment. It was cold and stark and the classrooms smelled funny. It was filled with machines that measured everything down to the smallest microbe. Everything we studied in botany and biology was dead and chopped up, a "slice and dice" learning method as opposed to that of learning from live plants in their wild environments—an educational experience with which I was more familiar.

I studied a variety of subjects that pertained to my work as an herbalist. My studies were interdisciplinary, unrelated to any particular degree

Study of Plants: Botanical Studies

If one were to define the education of an herbalist in academic terms, one could study these subjects:

Biology is the study of all organisms and how they work, from the smallest single cell organism to the complex human body. It is a perfect place to start.

Botany is the study of plants and how they work (this was my favorite course).

Taxonomy is the classification of plants and animals, determined by their similarities and the differences. If you think plant taxonomy is a boring subject, think again and start reading about past botanical expeditions that searched for plants from newly-discovered countries.

Plant Monographs are in-depth studies of particular plants, including their chemical breakdown as well as their historical uses and more. They are used by the scientific community to determine the uses of specific plants (medicinal or otherwise).

Ethnobotany is the study of plants and the environments in which they live and their traditional uses.

Horticulture programs train students in the art of growing plants for food and economic uses, such as flowering plants for gardens.

Sustainable Agriculture programs are currently taught in colleges. They teach how to grow plants without destroying the environment. I am so pleased to see this new development.

The Study of the Human Body: Medical Studies

Medical refers to medicine or the study of healing the body. Medical students are taught about the human body and how it works.

Anatomy is the study of the structure of our body, and **Physiology** is the study of the functions of the human body including the physical and chemical processes involved in its workings. **Pathology** is the study of what goes wrong in the body, or the study of the nature and cause of disease in the human body and how it affects the body.

Nutrition is the study of the nutritional qualities of food. A nutritionist is a person who studies nutrition and gives nutritional advice. In the New York State anyone can call themselves a nutritionist. To become a board-certified nutritionist, one must complete a certified program from an accredited institution. A **Dietician** is a person who is trained in nutrition, food science and diet planning. Institutes employ dieticians to plan their food services programs. The studies involve the chemistry of food and the breakdown of the nutritional content of the food into actual numbers. The labeling of the nutritional value of school lunch foods has become so strict and regimented that many schools choose not to participate in the farm to school programs.

Culinary programs teach food preparation. Usually they are completely separated from other disciplines even though their students are at the front line of nutrition (in that they actually prepare and cook the food that people eat).

Anthropology is the study of cultures as well as the study of the traditional uses of plants for medicines. This is integral to our understanding of botanical medicine.

Psychology and **sociology** are courses that try to understand the human psyche. These courses are essential to understanding the healing process. Anyone involved in the healing field finds very early on that there is a lot more to helping people get better than just using the right plant or the right drug.

Clinical experience refers to applying the knowledge gained in medical courses to actual cases. Since doctors and nurses are trained in the use of pharmaceutical drugs (not herbal plants), they do not have expertise in using botanical medicine; it is not part of their training. That is why doctors do not suggest herbal plants for medical conditions.

My Clinical Experience

So how did I get my clinical experience? I started using herbs on myself, my family, my animals and friends, but my greatest experiences came from treating uninsured kids in their twenties who had absolutely no access to the healthcare system. Until the Affordable Care Act came into being a short six years ago, a huge percentage of the population in this country had no access to any kind of health care. These kids refused to go to the ER and never went to doctors. They had no way to pay the exorbitant medical bills and fees, so unless it was life or death they didn't go. I treated these kids, FOR FREE, with herbal plants, while listening all the while to doctors and other experts as they ridiculed the healing attributes of plants like Echinacea on the nightly news and in magazines. As I helped these kids out I was appalled at a society that refused to provide decent and accessible healthcare to its future generation. I still get extremely upset when I think about the people involved in blocking access to healthcare. What message does this send, given that we live in one of the richest countries in the world? That healthcare is only available to the wealthy class. Healthcare is a birthright to all citizens living in the U.S.

As is the case, people became very smart and resourceful over time and started to use different types of healing modalities. In many cases they found that such alternative methods worked better than the healing methods sanctioned by our healthcare system. Now we must incorporate these different healing methods into our healthcare system in order to cause the cost of healthcare to go down and therefore become accessible to everyone.

Experiences of an Herbal Teacher

When I first started teaching about herbalism, the only places that felt comfortable enough to permit me to teach my subject were "new age" bookstores. I found this to be very funny, since using plants as medicine was as old as the earth itself. In the 1990s, I taught continuing education classes at the local, state-sponsored community college: there, I encountered the academic fear of teaching botanical medicine. Even today the prevailing attitude is to keep plants in the science department and not in the medical department. I received a call from a very fearful administrator just before my first herbal class started: she asked me not to talk about herbal plants but instead to talk about flowers. She thought that that would be safer and not a potential liability to the college. The college had a horticulture department, so a lecture on flowers wouldn't get anyone in trouble. I told her that all the plants I talk about have flowers.

My Apprenticeship Program

Teaching a seven month (spring, summer, fall) apprenticeship class was the best experience I have had involving people and the world of medicinal plants. The process of teaching about the natural world, gardening, the timing of nature and its bounty of plants was satisfying. This knowledge empowers people. It sets them on a different course giving them tools that they can use for the rest of their lives.

Certified Herbalist Programs from a University

At the moment there are no university-certified herbalist programs in the United States. We live in a society that holds the belief that you must have a degree from an accredited university before you can work and teach that subject. For instance, a medical degree enables you to work as a doctor. It also enables you to teach about medicine. On the other hand, there are no university-accredited programs for botanical medicine in this country at the moment. (You can get a degree in Chinese Botanical Medicine, which uses plants from China, but there is no degree program that uses plants from our country.) Although I have forty years' experience as an herbalist I cannot teach in a college setting. If you have an anthropology degree (they are allowed to teach about the history of the use of plant medicine but not their personal experience using herbs) or a nursing degree you can teach about herbs, but an experienced herbalist cannot teach in a college setting and get paid. That is the way in which the education system controls the health care system. This wasn't always the case. Homeopathic Colleges as well as Eclectic Colleges in the 19th and 20th century flourished but were closed in order to eliminate competition with sanctioned university medical institutions that emphasized drugs and surgery as opposed to botanicals and energy medicines.

First we were ignored, then we were ridiculed....

When I started learning about herbs, no one bothered us: we were basically ignored. People thought that I was quite eccentric, which was fine judging by what came later. As people started sharing their herbal success stories I noticed that the media started publishing and broadcasting stories that ridiculed herbs and the people who used them. It seems impossible to think of a world without internet but back then there was no access to alternative health information as there is today. We may be overwhelmed by the enormous amount of information online but at least we have access to that information.

A name-calling tactic that stands out to me refers to an herbal product known as "snake oil": the tactic involves calling the person who sells an herbal product a "snake oil salesman". These terms have evolved over the centuries to suggest that the herbal product for sale is fake, and that the person selling it is knowingly selling something that isn't that which is advertised. The terms have an interesting history. In the middle of the 1800s, Chinese workers who came to the U.S. to work on the Transcontinental Railroad brought with them their own medicines; one such medicine was made from the oil of the Chinese water snake. It was used successfully for inflammation and sore muscles. It was copied by many companies but it didn't have any of the ingredients that made the original snake oil work. "Patent Medicines" were being sold without any type of oversight and in 1906 the Pure Food and Drug Act was passed to protect the customer from fraudulent food, drugs, medicines and liquors. That was the precursor of the FDA.

Another popular name-calling tactic is to insult the intelligence of people who are using herbs. I have heard the expression: "Would you put an herb on a broken leg"? No one I know. People know when and where to use herbal plants and when to use the emergency room.

The media publishes many fear-based stories about people at risk of being jailed if they do not use conventional care for themselves or their children. There are many heartbreaking stories of parents unwilling to subject their children to any more chemotherapy or radiation. We need more information about what is actually happening in these cases as opposed to a quick soundbite.

Gone After by the Government

Under Governor Pataki's administration in 2000, New York State formed a committee called CAM which stands for Complementary and Alternative Medicine. My fellow herbalists and other alternative health care practitioners had become increasingly aware of increased government scrutiny. The government started focusing on the need to regulate the new healing methods that were proliferating across the United States since the 1960s. New York State is and was a very regulated state and was disciplining physicians by revoking their medical licenses if they used any type of alternative therapies, as well as if they failed to adhere to the "Standard of Care" that was the law. "Standard of Care" practice means that doctors can only use the techniques in which they are trained. In the United States, doctors are trained in the use of pharmaceutical drugs and surgery. (Which is the main reason many alternative healthcare people opposed the Affordable Care Act because they said (and rightly so) that nothing would change and people wanted so much more from their healthcare system.)

The CAM committee was formed to focus on regulatory and licensing issues. The people who worked on this project worked for the Department of the Health Regulatory Agency. Many of my fellow herbalists were visited by people from this "project". An official from the "Project" took my Herbal Apprenticeship course and after the course was finished I was advised not to teach anymore (which is wrong, since one can teach anything they wish in the U.S., as guaranteed by the right to free speech as stated in the Constitution). I just could not fathom why the government would waste any money investigating such a small-time herbalist and others who worked in the alternative health world. The government went after people individually: it was so frightening to the alternative health world that many people still refuse to talk about how they were harassed by different government officials and agencies. The New York State Education Department also got in the act of "health regulation" and threatened people who worked with different healing techniques. One of my herbal apprentice students was told by her visiting nurse agency that they knew she was taking my herbal apprenticeship course but that she was not allowed to use *anything* that she was learning in that course on her patients. I remember how incredibly upset she was when she told me. She was a young nurse and full of desire to help people.

The project and its staff was eliminated by Governor Spitzer's administration in 2007.

Follow the Money

There is a direct link between medical schools, physicians, hospitals, and government health institutions (such as FDA and NIH), and money from pharmaceutical companies. Pharmaceutical companies are the most profitable companies in the U.S. The amount of money they make is staggering.

Medical schools have a direct link to money from pharmaceutical companies through research grants; physicians receive direct payments or "gifts" (free trips) to use a certain drug or drugs. Medical papers are ghostwritten for doctors by the companies and published in prestigious medical journals such as the New England Journal of Medicine. One of the saddest cases of this came to my attention in 2008 through a congressional investigation. Dr. Joseph L. Biederman, a professor of psychiatry at Harvard Medical School and chief psychopharmacology at Mass General Hospital, was diagnosing children with bipolar disorder as young as two years old and was treating them with a variety of psychotropic drugs. It came to light that he was secretly being paid by the pharmaceutical companies who made those drugs. He took home 1.6 million in consulting fees (as did some of his colleagues). He and his colleagues still hold their positions. "The Truth about Drug Companies" by Marcia Angell, a former editor of the New England Journal of Medicine, details the influences of the drug companies on the way we practice medicine in this country.

Use the internet to learn about the fees that doctors receive as well as the campaign contributions that politicians receive in order to get a glimpse of the big picture of how medicine is affected by enormous sums of money.

"You are not going to believe this but the herbs worked!!!"

"Yes, I do believe it. I am so glad they worked for you," I say whenever I receive yet another happy phone call from an incredulous person. I have been doing this work for forty years and have witnessed the power of the plants. Remember: it is your birthright to know plants and the planet that they grow upon.

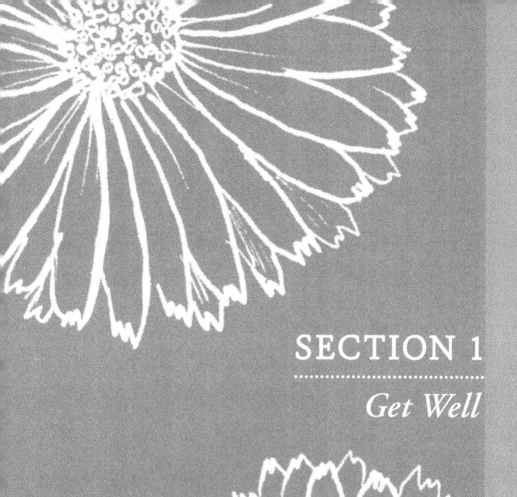

SECTION 1

·························

Get Well

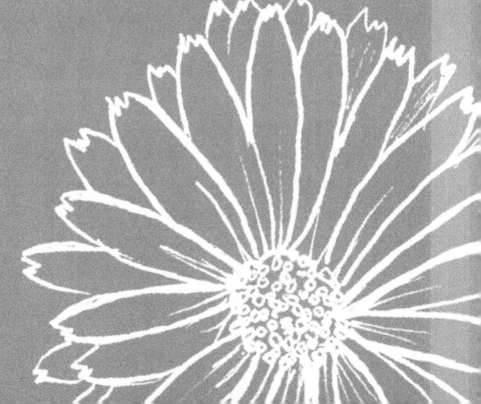

Chapter 1

INTRODUCTION

"I was sitting in front of my TV, wrapped in blankets, struggling to shake an awful Flu Bug that was orbiting my world. Everyone seemed to have "It" or a variation of "It". My local PBS TV station aired a program about the Flu and the news anchor interviewed 2 people on what they did to avoid coming down with the flu. Each said that they take Echinacea and orange juice when they feel a cold or flu coming on. The consensus was that there wasn't anything you could do, I groaned, knowing what was coming next. Sure enough, the next interview was with a MD stating that Echinacea isn't effective at all, but if it makes you feel like you are doing something, go ahead and take it; after all, the power of placebo is very effective. He followed with the well worn remark about how the studies aren't really there and they are inconclusive, blah, blah, blah."

I wrote those words over a decade ago for a magazine article titled "What the Local Herbalist does when faced was the flu." I was totally frustrated with the lack of knowledge in our society about what to do when faced with the latest variation of winter ills. And I am not just talking about herbal knowledge. Although there are myriad actions to take when "coming down with something", if you went into a drugstore in the U.S. you would find few options. This is not the case in other countries. In Europe the apothecaries are filled with all sorts of remedies for colds and the flu, particularly herbal remedies. When I was in Austria I picked up a bottle of an herbal digestion tonic at the local grocery store. The herbal tonic *Gurktaler Alpenkrauter* contains a combination of 59 different plants and has been made from the same recipe for hundreds of years. It works just as well today as it did then.

I use herbal plants to help alleviate symptoms and move through the occasional winter illness. Just as we need food to feed and nourish our bodies, the use of herbal plants helps correct the imbalance caused by a cold or flu in the body. The use of herbal plants also helps us from becoming sick. One of the biggest concerns of grandparents is catching the latest 'bug' from their grandchildren. Herbs can help keep our immune system strong so that we are not susceptible to every germ that comes our way. I am in the presence of five grandchildren and am exposed to just about everything on a daily basis.

The plants, herbal preparations, and herbal techniques in this book are the ones I have been using for myself, my family and my clients. They are tried and true, gleaned from over 30 years' worth of experience as an herbalist. I am comfortable with the use of these plants. They work well. I grow most of the plants I use. I also "wildcraft", or harvest from the wild, many of the plants that I talk about in this book.

After living all over the country, I now live in the Adirondacks—a mountainous area in the northeast corner of New York State. When I moved this far north I wasn't certain of the actual growing season. It seemed quite short. I am closer to Montreal, Canada than to New York City. (For all the gardeners out there, I am in zone 4.) I made it my business to learn about what grew around me. I am still amazed by the wealth and abundance of plants that grow here. In fact, so many wild plants that I talk about in this book are considered pesky weeds, and they positively thrive in my neck of the woods. In the Plant Section I have provided detailed growing information for most of the plants that I talk about in the book.

Local Food, Local Herbs

Using local plants means that the plants are as fresh as can be, and just like eating local food using local herbs makes a huge difference. Local herbal plants are the right medicine for the people who live around them. Because you have grown or wildcraft the herbal plants yourself, you know exactly what you are using (and gain, too, the enormous satisfaction of gardening). Growing and harvesting the plants yourself creates a sense of satisfaction and security all through the year. In every area of the country there are herb farm-

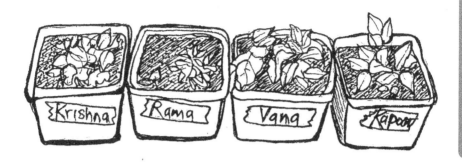

ers selling high quality herbs and herb plants, so don't let the fact that you aren't a gardener deter you from using herbal remedies.

The herbal plants and preparations in this book are not the only plants and preparations out there: far from it. They are the plants that work for me. (I tell my students that I am in a "plant rut" because I always seem to use the same plants.)

Several years ago I tried growing several species of holy basil or tulsi. I noticed that tulsi had become a well-liked herbal plant. It comes from the Ayurvedic tradition which hails from India. Of the four species I found that the Kapoor species flourished in my northern gardens and now I harvest more tulsi than any other plant. I was surprised by how happy and hearty the plant turned out to be in Upstate New York. The experiment was well worth it. I encourage you to explore the wonder of the plant kingdom. Start by harvesting the plants in your garden. So many people grow culinary herbs in their gardens but never harvest them for later use. Many culinary herbs are also considered medicinal plants.

Just as people are unique, the plants and preparations that work for different individuals are unique as well. There are ancient healing traditions all over the world that use plants as medicines. I suggest reading about different cultures' use of herbal plants. Hopefully this book will be a starting point in discovering the world of healing plants for yourself.

How herbal plants work for colds and the flu

Herbs prevent illness from taking hold. They help the body not become as sick. They help the body recover faster from an illness. They ease symptoms. They enable you to stay well and not become reinfected.

Everyday Herbal Nutrition

My favorite category of herbs is that which contains the plants that keep us healthy and that can be taken every day. They work as insurance for good health, loaded with vitamins, minerals and other substances that keep us feeling strong and healthy. These herbs are referred to as tonics. Sometimes people feel that it is only a matter of time before they succumb to the latest illness. It doesn't have to be that way. Drinking lots of water and nutritional herbal teas, using nutritional herbal powders, getting extra sleep and basically slowing down can help us maintain our healthy immune system when faced with an unhealthy environment. These plants work as "preventatives" in addition to keeping us healthy.

Herbal Preventatives

These herbs work by providing the body with the extra nutrients and specific substances it needs to fight off an acute illness or a "state of imbalance" (how the herbalist describes the feeling that "you aren't right: you're not sick, but you're not your regular self"). These plants work as "immune stimulators"—that is, they work by boosting the immune system's actions to fight off infections and to keep the body well. For example, the Echinacea plant boosts the production of white blood cells in the body, thereby helping the body fight off an incoming infection. Elderberry works in a similar manner. These plants work well during the beginning of an imbalance as preventatives. They also work as an extra insurance health boost when people are exposed to illness. These preventative plants are especially useful for people who work in the public realm.

Not As Sick, Recover Faster

Herbal plants do not cure colds or the flu, but they help your immune system cope with the illness so that you do not become as sick as you might have had you done nothing at all. Using herbs to alleviate the symptoms helps the body cope with the illness so that you will not be as adversely affected by the illness.

Ease of symptoms

Herbs help the body cope with cold and flu symptoms. The extra nutrients in the herbs nourish and protect the body. The root of the marshmallow plant works as a demulcent. The action of a demulcent plant coats and sooths mucous membranes like the lining of the lungs, sinuses and intestines. Drinking a decoction of marshmallow root helps soothe the respiratory tract. This helps the body move through the illness. It eases the severity of the illness so that you are not as sick; you get better faster and stay better.

Comfort

Herbal plants ease the symptoms of an illness so that the body can rest better. This is so important because we heal when we rest and sleep. Sometimes all it takes is a hot cup of herbal tea to bring comfort to an ailing person.

Calming

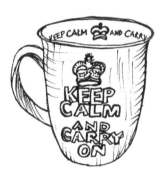

Herbs that contain substances that help your body relax and slow down are called nervines. Herbs that calm and sedate create a better environment for getting well. Remember the feeling of being sick, and how tired you can become of feeling sick. In our society we are not used to being anything less than busy, busy, busy people. Chamomile tea is calming to both the nervous and digestive systems and is a wonderful tool to calm a sick child.

Stay well

Recently, I have noticed a trend: many people seem to not be able to "stay better" after an illness. They seem to be vulnerable to the next "bug" right after they have recovered from the first. This is so discouraging. Herbal plants can help us stay healthy. Utilizing nutritional herbs after an illness helps restore the body to health and stay that way.

The time you spend taking care of yourself in the beginning of an imbalance will pay off in the end.

Using herbal plants to chase away the illness is an action game. But it is worth the effort. Start using herbal remedies as soon as possible.

Share the Knowledge

Teach people in your household what to do in case you, the caretaker, gets sick. I learned this the hard way when I succumbed to the flu one winter and learned that no one in my household had any idea how to make a simple herbal infusion.

Stock Up Before Cold Season

Keep well-labeled herbal teas, capsules and tinctures in the house before the cold/flu season arrives. When you become sick (which is usually at 9 pm on a Sunday night) you do not feel like mixing up herbal formulas, let alone driving across town to purchase them (where you might not even find what you are looking for).

Keep Records

Use a small notebook to write down what works for you and your family. I suggest taking notes right in this book. Write down each person's symptoms and the names of the herbs that worked for them. No one wants to revisit the times they were sick, and that lack of memory seems to lead us to forget what herbs helped us get better. So record what you took and why—you will be happy that you took the time.

In my family, my son and daughter were sick in different ways. My son was sick as a child much more so than my daughter. His illnesses seemed to linger, and I found that using stimulant herbs in his herbal remedies (such as the addition of cayenne in cold capsules) was important in order to get him better.

My daughter, on the other hand, would just go to bed and not want to be bothered at all. So much of my experience comes from trying different herbs and recording what worked with my family and friends. I still look at those three-ring notebooks of my herbal adventures with great fondness.

Green Pills or Yellow Pills

My kids grew up with herbal medicine. When they went away to college, I realized that they had figured out the whole herbal healing system. They used to call me up and have me send them the green pills or the yellow pills. They used the green caps when they were well and the yellow caps when they were coming down with something. It was that simple.

The green capsules contain herbs that are very high in nutrition: nettles, oats, alfalfa, spirilina, dandelion leaf, horsetail. They used them as someone would use vitamins pills, extra insurance for their health.

The yellow capsules contain strong anti microbial herbs "specific" for colds and flus: Goldenseal, Myrrh, Marshmallow Root, Echinacea root, Cayenne. They are a one stop shopping type of herbal remedy for cold or flu symptoms. Taken at the onset of the illness they usually worked to shorten up the duration of what ailed them.

"I got better but it wasn't the herbs"

I cannot tell you how many times I have heard this comment throughout my years as an herbalist. Herbal medicine is simple and it works. Here in lies the problem: people think that simple doesn't work. **It does.**

Simple Works

If the only thing you learn from this book is how to make a cup of medicinal herbal tea, that would be the most important skill over all, and the most helpful, not just for your sake but for everyone around you. A cup of tonifying herbal tea not only helps our bodies get better but brings immeasurable comfort to us and to those whom we are helping. Never, ever think that a cup of tea is too simple to help, on the contrary, it is the most powerful tool we can use for ourselves and the people around us.

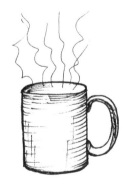

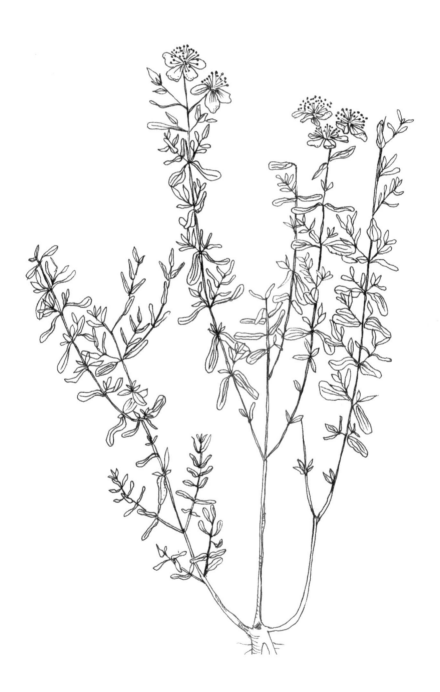

Chapter 2

USING THE
WHOLE PLANT

The best way to use plants for food and medicine is to use the whole plant in the simplest way possible. A tea or infusion of dried leaves or a decoction of roots is simple. Grinding up the leaves or roots and ingesting the powder in a capsule or drink is simple. (Creating an alcohol tincture or vinegar extract would be a little more complicated.) Keep the preparation simple and utilize the whole plant.

Plants contain hundreds of constituents that work together in the body to help nourish and heal it. We do not know everything there is to know about the way in which plants can help us. Every day I read an article about the way plants do what they do. The science of botany is an ongoing exploration of new insights about the plant kingdom.

The best example of using the whole plant for optimal healing properties is playing out in almost every state in the union. The battle to legalize the marijuana plant has been going on for decades. In the 1930s, immediately after prohibition law was repealed, the marijuana plant was declared illegal. Today it is still classified as a schedule one drug and not as a plant. Cannabis or marijuana has been used for centuries as medicine. In the 1980s, pharmaceutical companies produced a drug from the marijuana plant called Marinol. It was marketed as a drug to help with the nausea caused by chemotherapy. The drug contains a synthesized (manmade) form of THC, which is only one of the many hundreds of constituents contained in the Cannabis plant. According to the pharmaceutical company, the THC constituent was the medicinal component of the plant and was responsible for the nausea relief that people experienced when they smoked the marijuana plant after receiving chemotherapy. The drug Marinol did not work as promised. THC is also responsible for the "high", or altered mindset, that people experience when using the plant. Currently, we hear about another Cannabis constituent, CBD. This constituent is now being promoted as the medicinal part of the plant as opposed to the THC. CBD oil preparations are readily available to the consumer as opposed to medical marijuana preparations which are highly regulated.

A friend that uses medical marijuana for severe chronic pain needs a tincture preparation that contains a much larger percentage of the THC constituent than the CBD constituent for relief of her pain.

The cannabis plant contains hundreds of constituents, so isolating just one constituent and declaring it to be the part of the plant that works is short sighted.

Several years ago, companies started selling "standardized extract" versions of herbal plants. The supplements were advertised as containing the correct amount of a constituent, thus making the product effective. These standardized extract preparations were touted as the answer to using herbs because finally one could measure "one" of the plant's medicinal components. The companies fostered the perception that the plant alone wasn't good enough— that herbal plants weren't strong enough. They propagated the idea that you needed to change the plant's form, turning it into a form more like a drug preparation. This makes for good sales but it wasn't necessary, because using the whole plant works.

Plants contain hundreds of constituents that work together in the body to help heal. We do not know all of what the plants contain nor how the different constituents work together to form a medicine that works without harm. Making a product or a pharmaceutical drug out of just one plant constituent and offering it in a mega dose is like using a jackhammer rather than a pushpin to solve a health problem. It is neither necessary nor wise.

Chapter 3

RIGHT PLANT,
RIGHT PREPARATION,
RIGHT DOSAGE:
HOW TO USE THE BOOK

The trick to using herbal plants for healing is to figure out what plant or plants are the best for your health issue. The next step is to pick the right preparation for the herbal plant that you are using. Lastly, you need to figure how much to take, or determine the dosage, of that herbal preparation to get better.

Right Plant

Fortunately for us, the herbs for cold and flu conditions are tried and true. These plants have been used for thousands of years to help the body rid itself of the occasional illness.

These plants have time and empirical knowledge on their side. For instance, when using an herb such as yarrow blossoms for cold or flu-like illness, the herbs that are anti-viral are usually anti-bacterial and anti-fungal as well. They are called anti-microbial herbs. As such, they work whether or not you have a cold or the flu. In the **Language of Herbalism** section I have listed the different actions of the plants. For instance, marshmallow root is a demulcent which means that it soothes and protects the mucous membranes of the body.

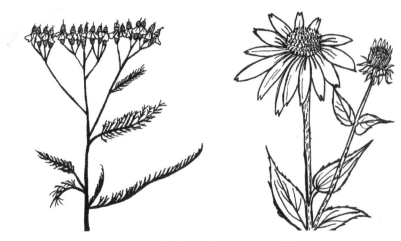

Yarrow (left), Echinacea (right)

Herbal plants work for the whole body, body system, part of that body system and for particular cold/flu symptoms. Yarrow and catnip helps the whole body. Marshmallow root helps the upper and lower respiratory system. Sage, the ordinary culinary herb, works specifically on the throat—it is a "specific" for a sore throat. Many plants are called 'specifics' when they help remedy certain symptoms of a cold/flu.

When we are sick with the common cold or the flu, our respiratory, digestive, and nervous systems seem to be affected most. But the respiratory system seems to get the brunt of it.

I talk in detail about the herbs that are indicated for these four systems in the **Respiratory, Digestive, Nervous** and **Immune System** sections. Read about the actions of these particular body systems and the corresponding herbal plants that help alleviate the symptoms associated with the particular body symptom.

For instance, coughing is a symptom of a respiratory imbalance. There are different types of coughs. I have listed the different plants and their actions for the different types of coughs. It is important to move the mucous out of the lungs so the use of an expectorant herb is indicated. Sometimes the use of an anti-tussive is indicated when the cough is annoying rather than useful for the body. Anti-tussives calm the coughing reflex which helps a person get the rest they need to get well.

If you are in a hurry, please refer to the **Symptoms** section: here, symptoms are listed alongside the specific herbs and herbal preparations that are used for the symptoms you are experiencing. After that, you can look up related recipes in the **Herbal Recipe** section. Do not become overwhelmed by the many choices. I give a variety of options because the plants work that way and you might have different herbs on hand (especially if you have an herbal garden). Determine what works best for you and then turn to the **Preparation** section for directions on how to make the recipes.

I have underlined the plants that have a history of being specific for particular problems. You will usually need just one or two preparations. By all means, do not forget to use herbs for external applications, too.

Right Preparation

When you figure out what plant you want to use, then you need to prepare it properly so that you receive the maximum benefits of the plant. Originally, I planned on writing a book that was just an illustrated version of the proper way to prepare herbal plants. But I became concerned about the lack of solid information about how to properly prepare herbal plants for medicinal use. Millions of people are using medicinal herbs, and botanical medicine is going to be the future of medicine because that is what people want.

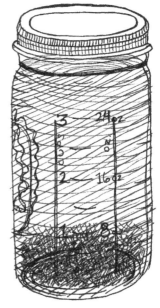

I have two major issues with improper herbal preparation. Both regard the creation of water-based preparations. The first is about making a tea or infusion using leaves. The cup of tea is usually not covered when it is steeping, and is not steeped for a substantial amount of time.

Covering a cup of steeping herbal tea ensures that the voluble oils do not escape through the steam. Steeping the herb tea for at least thirty minutes ensures that you are getting the constituents needed for the health benefits. It is a mystery to me why the steeping times in so many herbal books are only five minutes or so. I rarely see information about placing a cover on the tea while it is steeping.

The second issue that concerns me about improper herbal preparation involves the way in which roots are prepared. Roots are strong and dense. They need to be prepared differently than leaves and flowers. They need to be simmered in water on the stove for 20 minutes to release their healing benefits. They can also be used again. It is such a waste to steep them in hot water for 5 minutes. It is a waste of the plant's power when the roots aren't prepared properly.

The preparation section contains illustrated, detailed information about how to prepare herbal plants to maximize their healing benefits. All the important preparations are thoroughly covered, as well as bone broths and turmeric milk. Refer to the **Children's Section** for tips on giving herbal preparations to children.

Make what you will actually use

The preparations you prepare should fit your lifestyle and should be prepared in quantities that you plan to actually use. Herbal capsules and tinctures are much easier to take on the run. If you have a hard time slowing down, make sure you have a supply of herbs in capsule and tincture form in your medicine cabinet **before** you get sick. I make a large supply of Cold Capsules and Yellow Pills in the fall. Although a cup of hot herbal tea is very healing, it's not the preparation for you if you won't spend the time to make it. Sometimes getting sick is the only time people slow down enough to welcome such a cup of healing tea as they finally lie down to rest.

Taste is important

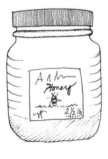

Honey

When my son was a small boy, I decided after reading all these herbal books that horehound was the right herb for whatever ailed him. He loved being sick and hanging out at home—lying on the couch, watching TV, and missing school. But I was new to the world of healing plants at the time and did not understand how to make herbs palatable.

I knew that horehound had a bitter and acrid taste: all the old herbals had recipes that encouraged the creation of horehound candy or otherwise used a lot of sugar in their preparations. I got the idea to make horehound candy (which is very strange as I never used white sugar for anything). I bought a candy thermometer and made the horehound candy to give my son pieces from time to time. Surprisingly, he got better: I was amazed how well the horehound worked. Weeks later, I would still find pieces of horehound candy stuck to the walls behind the radiator, stuck to the bottom of the couch, and hidden in places where I couldn't see them.

Since that time, I have learned to disguise the taste of so many strong herbs with other good-tasting herbs or by making more palatable syrup preparations. I have found that adults love elderberry syrup just as much as kids do. I have also learned to make very small amounts of herbal recipes before I commit to making large quantities, just to be sure that I get the flavor right.

Right Dosages

After determining the right plants and their preparation, it is time to figure out what dosage you need. Posology is a fancy term for the art of dosaging. Please check out the **Posology** section for guidelines for all ages. The correct dosage depends on the plants, the preparation and the person. The trick is to take enough of the herb for the proper amount of time in order to alleviate your symptoms or condition. Take an herbal mixture slowly at first. Try out a decoction or an herbal infusion and wait and see how you feel. Everyone reacts to herbs differently. Some people are very sensitive to anything they ingest. These people usually do well with medicinal herbs insofar as they are habituated to listening to their bodies. I have found that most people possess an innate wisdom when it comes to choosing the right plants, preparations, and how much they should take and for how long.

Considering that we do not have herbalists in this country to tell us what to do (currently there are no certified herbal programs in the U.S., and doctors and nurses receive no training in herbal medicine), I think people are doing extremely well by themselves. Therein lies another important point about using medicinal plants: they are safe. Compare the safety record of herbal plants to pharmaceutical drugs. The numbers tell the story.

People run the gamut when it comes to using herbal preparations. I know people who have bought into the fear-mongering propagated by news stations so much that they are too afraid to drink a cup of chamomile tea. On the other hand, some people have been convinced by aggressive marketing campaigns that the only plant preparations worth taking are essential oils. These people use them externally and internally (it is illegal to use essential oils internally in the U.S.) with very little knowledge of the strength of such preparations and their effects on and in the body.

More is not better nor necessary

It is indeed human nature to be tempted to take a whole lot of a preparation if you find something that works. Some might think that if one cup of an herbal infusion works, then *four* cups should work even better. Not so! It is not the case that "a lot" is better than "a little". But you still need to take enough of the herbal preparation to do the job.

Since my daughter grew up with access to large quantities of herbs and herbal preparations, she doesn't think about how much is too much when preparing herbs. I have watched my daughter (now an adult) make a quart of catnip infusion with a half cup of catnip, and I've also watched her take a quarter cup of echinacea tincture at a time. But there is no need to take too much: in my experience, the dosage guidelines in the Posology section work well for most people. As you use herbs you will figure out what works for you and your family.

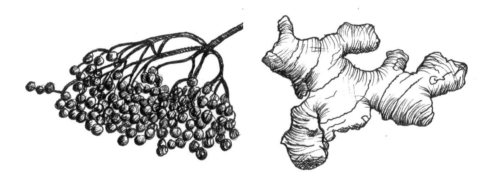

Elderberries (left), Ginger Root (right)

16

Chapter 4

HERBS FOR OUTSIDE
OF THE BODY

The use of herbs on the outside of the body is just as important as using herbs internally: in fact, using herbs externally can sometimes be the most effective way to deal with the symptoms of an illness. Combined with the healing power of herbal plants, water in all its forms—steam, ice, in hot and cold packs, and in submersion baths—is so helpful and comforting when struggling through an illness.

Sinus Steam

I first recognized the importance of the external use of herbs upon noticing the rising popularity of one of my herbal products, Sinus Steam. I sell more of my Sinus Steam mixture than any other herbal mixture. Steaming the sinuses with herbal steam is so effective for all types of respiratory imbalances and headaches of all sorts (not to mention as a treatment for facial skin). I listened to so many complaints from students and family members about

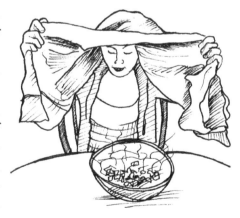

the difficulties of using neti pots that I developed an alternative method of cleaning the large sinus cavities and nasal passages. The herbal steam seems to penetrate much better than does a neti pot and has the added benefit of assisting the lungs as well.

Herbal Bathing

Another "outside" preparation is herbal bathing. I use this treatment extensively. Years ago, I made a cup of boneset infusion for my kids who were sick with the flu. I had not tasted boneset myself at that time as I was new to the world of plants, but I had read about its incredible healing powers when used for the flu. Boneset is the premier herb for relieving the symptoms of the flu, and it works wonders when it comes to alleviating the "achy bones" feeling that sometimes comes with a viral illness. But to say that boneset tea is bitter would be an understatement: I realized that there was no way I could serve such a bitter-tasting tea to my kids. As a solution, I put the tea into a hot bath with my kids. I felt that it defiantly helped. From then on, I was hooked on bathing with herbal teas. I now favor catnip and yarrow as my favorite bath herbs.

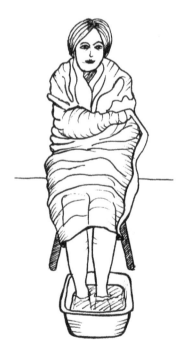 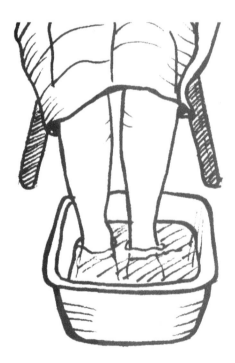

A chamomile bath helps the body to relax and get the sleep that it needs to heal. The diaphoretic actions of the herbs I use in my herbal baths help move the cold/flu out of the body. I used to give my children yarrow baths when they were sick, and after the baths I would wrap them up in lots of blankets to "sweat" out their colds.

Herbal foot baths are great in pinch when you do not feel like taking a whole bath. Nowadays, many people do not have bathtubs or never use them if they do. Many students are quite skeptical when I suggest that soaking in an herbal bath is similar to soaking in a big pot of herbal tea—and just as effective as drinking it. I consider herbal bathing to fall into my category of "Just shut up and do it, then talk to me": you might not expect it, but herbal bathing heals the body in a wonderful way.

Hydrotherapy

Hydrotherapy, or using water in all forms to treat illnesses, has long been used as a healing method. "Taking the waters" is a time-honored method of restoring and maintaining health. I live close by to many natural mineral springs in Upstate New York, the most famous of which are the many natural springs of Saratoga Springs. The healing properties of the many different springs were well-known to the American Indians, who later introduced them to the settlers. Over time, a health and spa industry would form about the mineral waters of Saratoga. Many of my friends from Saratoga Springs grew up drinking the mineral waters from the different springs that exist all over the city. They know all the city's springs and would gladly stick their heads under a spring fountain spout for a drink. I am not there yet.

Poultices

Applying herbs directly to the skin is a time-honored tradition and it works. Poultices are sometimes called plasters (such as in mustard plaster), fomentations, or compresses. Poultices can be directly applied to the skin: for instance, I have put a sliced onion atop bruises and bee stings. Likewise, a warm onion poultice to the chest will help dissipate congestion. For headaches, a ginger poultice can work wonders.

Eye Wash

An herbal eyewash helps alleviate symptoms of pink eye and its variations. For centuries, people have used glass eye cups to bath the eye with herbal solutions. Bathing the eyes with a cup of an herbal solution is faster, easier, and more effective than trying to pour saline from a plastic bottle into the eyes. A grandmother of a friend used to use a large spoon to rinse out the eyes. In fact, many people grew up bathing their eyes with boric acid.

Gargling

Gargling is a lost art. I was encouraged to gargle with warm saltwater when I was a kid; it was a tradition when dealing with a sore throat. As a kid, I thought that it was disgusting: the saltwater tasted awful and the whole procedure was gross. But gargling with sage tea is a very effective way to cure a sore throat. The healing properties of the herb get right where they need to be. Gargling big and noisy is the way to go: just wrap a towel around your neck and go at it! Last winter, my daughter was so sick of dealing with a sore throat that she even gargled with cayenne tea. It worked, but she said it was very intense. There is no need for such extreme measures. Sage tea tastes fine: in fact, it has a long history of medicinal uses beyond its culinary functions. (It does not taste like a turkey dinner!) I receive so many skeptical looks when I suggest that sage teas can taste amazing. I consider the use of sage tea for sore throats as another member of my "Just shut up and do it" category.

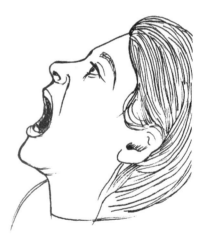

Sprays for Throat and Nose

Just like gargling, spraying herbal teas or diluted herbal tinctures down the throat can help alleviate the pain of a sore throat. To deliver a spray, use a small spray bottle to deliver the liquid to the throat with the aim of hitting the tonsils. Children like this herbal preparation. Often, I create a good-tasting herbal tea and put it into a spray bottle for my grandson: he then happily squirts the mixture into his mouth, coating his tonsils. I have noticed that anything that you do for children is very popular for adults as well. I use a nasal bottle in the same way.

Cold Sores

Apply a topical licorice tincture to cold sores (such as those that many people experience when they get sick) in order to prevent them from getting bigger and to make them go away faster. Licorice tinctures taste good, too!

Warm Mist Humidifiers

Many people heat their homes with wood stoves where I live. After several months of being exposed to this very drying type of heat, many people begin to develop dry sinuses. Dry sinuses can easily lead to the development of a sinus or lung infection. For this reason, make sure to add humidity to the house in the winter.

When used nightly, a warm mist humidifier helps the body cope with the dry air of winter heating systems. But humidifiers also provide essential relief to those struggling with respiratory illnesses. When dealing with an illness, make sure to use a *warm* air humidifier (as cold air humidifiers do not work at all). Buy one for every bedroom—not just for the children's room. I go through about one every two years as I use it nightly during the winter season. Humidifiers come apart and are easy to clean. Of course, it is important to clean them on a regular basis.

Heating Pads

I find that heating pads work to soothe many bodily aches. They help comfort sore throats, sore chests, and aching heads. When my son struggled with earaches, I would heat up kosher salt in a cast iron pan on the stove to fill tube socks (remember tube socks?) And place them on his ears to help with the pain. There are many different types of heating pads that one can purchase. You can find directions to make your own microwavable heating pads in the **Preparation** section. When sick with a cough, a heating pad placed on the chest will comfort children quite a lot.

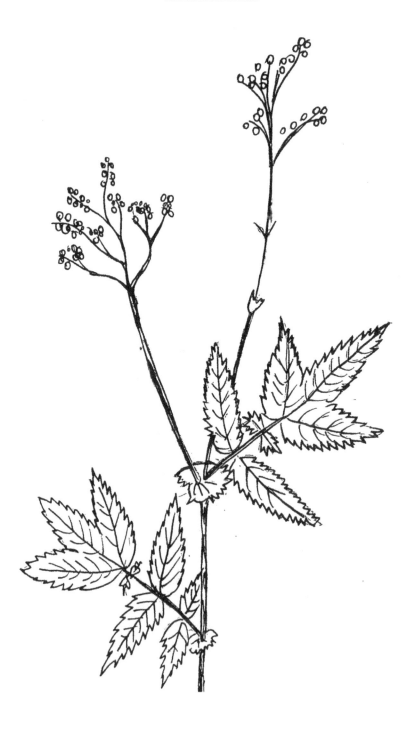

Chapter 5

POSOLOGY

Posology is the fancy term for the art of determining how much of an herbal preparation one needs to take to get well. Figuring out the right medicinal dosage is both an art and a science. General guidelines established centuries ago exist for each type of herbal preparation. After years of watching people use herbs, I think that these guidelines (stated at the end of the chapter) are generally effective. As with all things that pertain to the art of healing, what is considered "normal" is wide indeed.

Listen to your body

Since bodies are different, dosing needs are different, too. If you are sensitive to pharmaceutical drugs or even aspirin, then you should take a lower dosage of an herbal preparation than what is recommended. I have found that people who are sensitive to pharmaceutical drugs do well with herbal preparations. Start off slowly and increase your consumption. Feel how your body reacts. When taking herbs to help the body relax (such as chamomile), the effects can be felt right away. It is more difficult to judge the effectiveness of other types of herbal preparations.

Dosage is determined by weight

Dosage is based on the weight of an individual. An "adult weight" is considered to be about 150 lbs. Keep this in mind when determining how much of an herbal preparation to give to adults, teenagers, and children because they will either weigh less or more depending on the individual.

Take enough to do the job

Take enough of an herbal preparation to do the job but not so much that the body experiences a reaction or gets overstimulated. Redeveloping the symptoms that you are trying to eliminate can be a side effect of using the wrong herb or of using too high of a dosage. As you get better, the dosage should be reduced until you no longer need to take anything at all. Paying attention to the body is important: if symptoms begin to worsen, resume taking the herbs. Herbs are not like pharmaceutical drugs and dietary supplements: they are not meant to be taken forever. They do their job and the body heals. This is especially the case when dealing with acute conditions such as a cold or the flu.

Dosage Dependent

Some herbs, like echinacea, can be taken in much larger amounts than suggested. Such herbs are considered to be "dosage dependent", meaning that they need to be taken in sufficient quantities so that they can work in the body. In the case of Echinacea, the dosage for an Echinacea tincture preparation is higher than normally suggested: ½ to 1 tsp of tincture, up to four times a day, when trying to shake a cold.

Acute and Chronic Tonic Dosages

It is recommended to use a higher dosage when using herbs for an acute condition such as a cold or flu. Chronic conditions require a reduced dosage. If using herbs for a wellness tonic, it is recommended that you use even less of a dosage.

Be consistent: Figure out a strategy and stick to it

It is important to commit to taking the herbs and for a sufficient period of time so that the herbs have a chance to work in the body. It is important to maintain the levels of the medicinal herbs in the body, so taking the herbal preparations every day, and two to three times a day, is an effective strategy when using herbs to overcome an illness.

I think that many people go wrong when they fail to take herbal preparations on a consistent basis. They either do not take the herbs on a regular basis during their illness or stop taking them the minute they feel some kind of improvement. Herbal plants work as tonics in the body and the body's various systems; they help move the illness out of the body and keep the body from becoming reinfected. If you do not take them regularly when sick, they won't be able to help you. People tend to become tired of drinking their herbal preparations, steaming their sinuses, taking detoxing baths, and—most of all—slowing down and staying in bed. I'm actually talking about my own behavior: by day five, I am sick of doing anything and am most of all sick of being sick. But if you continue to comply with your herbal regimen, you will receive the biggest benefit of all: you will get better faster and will not get sick again soon after healing. I have met so many people who spend the entire winter catching one illness after another. They do not feel good for an entire winter season. The immune system wears down if the body remains in such an imbalanced state. Make the effort to get well. Make the commitment to take your medicinal herbs so that you can get well and stay well.

Ease of Preparation

Using herbs to get well is an action game. Taking a pill or capsule or even an herbal tincture is much easier than taking the time to make a cup of tea. Have several different types of herbal preparations available to you in your medicine cabinet in case you do not feel like making an infusion. Since I know that I am prone to sinus problems, I keep capsules of a goldenseal blend as well as goldenseal pills and goldenseal tinctures in case I need them. Although goldenseal is a very strong herb (it is intensely bitter, and not my favorite thing to drink), I know that it is the herb that works for me. But in a pinch, I will draw from my goldenseal supply gladly. I seem to run out of my cold capsules frequently. I supply my kids and their families with herbs so it seems that whatever I need the cold caps, I find that I have given away my supply. (Yet no one has ever taken my goldenseal tincture— I wonder why?)

Different Preparations, Different Dosages

You can drink several cups of water-based infusions and decoctions daily, but use only a fraction of that amount when using alcohol-based tinctures. Take 1-2 pills and capsules several times a day. It is important to figure out what works for you when deciding what preparation to take. Water-based preparations can be very healing during the first stages of an illness, but as you resume your busy lifestyle later on, pills or a tincture might be the way to go. By switching, you are still taking your herbs. It's easy to take a bottle of tincture or capsules to work or to keep a second bottle of tincture at work so that you remember to take your herbs.

Tincture Drops?

If you examine the suggested dosages on the backs of most herbal tincture bottles you will see that the suggested dosage amount is measured in drops. They suggest 30-60 drops several times a day. Thirty drops approximates ¼ teaspoon. I use teaspoon and tablespoon measurements because people are more familiar with these measurements and have the measuring spoons on hand. I suggest measuring out the drops that you are taking into a teaspoon the first time you take an herbal tincture in order to get an idea of how much you will need to take. It is a lot easier to take a spoonful of tincture then to spend all that time measuring out drops every time you take your tincture. Many herbal books suggest 1 to 2 droppers' worth. But it is impossible to measure out a full dropper's worth from a 1 oz. bottle. Most herbal tincture bottles found in stores are 1 oz. bottles. A regular squirt from a dropper is equal to about ¼ teaspoon. A full dropper, or two squirts, is about ½ of a teaspoon. Many of the herbal books contain metric measurements because they originate from Europe. Please refer to the conversion charts in the index of the book to figure out the proper dosages.

My Favorite Preparations: Syrups

Although syrup-making takes more time initially, the payoff is that the preparation you have made will last for a month or so. With five grandchildren I always keep a bottle of elderberry syrup in my refrigerator, along with garlic honey infusion. These are my staples for winter season.

Essential Oil Preparations

It is sad to see the lack of proper information when it comes to the popular preparation of essential oils. I have fielded so many questions about what to do with all the bottles of unused essential oil blends on people's shelves. Essential oils are very strong and should only be mixed with a carrier oil (a fixed oil such as olive or almond oil) to be used properly. Most people are confused about whether or not they have a bottle of an essential oil blend mixed with a carrier oil or a bottle of the straight essential oil itself. The dosage for straight essential oil is one to two drops. In this country, essential oils are only to be used externally or topically. I know that many people use essential oils internally as well without much education in how they work in the body. I urge caution when it comes to using such a strong plant preparation (especially with children). I have heard so many stories about people not feeling well after using essential oils. After asking further questions, it usually seems to be the case that the person did not realize how strong essential oils are, they also misjudged the dosage, and did not know how to use the essential oil preparation properly.

U.S.A. versus U.K.

I have been reading herbal books from the United Kingdom for years. As in most of the world, the study and practice of herbalism is a long-standing tradition in England. The dosages for herbal preparations are vastly different than those you would find here in the United States. For instance, it is common for their directions to prepare an herbal infusion to require 1 oz. dried herbs to one pint water, which translates to ½ - 1 cup dried herbs to 2 cups water. In the U.S., we use 2 teaspoons herbs to 2 cups water. They also suggest a dosage of 1-2 cups daily. Thus, books from the U.K. recommend a much higher dose of herbs than the standard dose recommended in texts from the United States.

It is also important to know that tincture bottles found in the U.K. are bigger than U.S. standard bottles (which are 1 oz. bottles). If you are using a normal tincture dose, you will find that the 1 oz. bottle goes quickly. To further distinguish the two, an English dosage is measured differently as well: in the U.K., tinctures are administered by teaspoons or tablespoons; in the U.S., tincture intake is measured in drops.

Fear Factor

It is a mystery to me that people who do not question their pharmaceutical drug intake can be very afraid of overdosing on herbal formulas. If you are nervous about taking herbal remedies, it is important to start slow and with a small dosage. If you feel like you have taken too much, just drink several glasses of water to flush out the system.

Too many cups of coffee

When I ask the question, "What are two herbs that Americans are addicted to?" most people know to answer "tobacco", but few figure out that the other and much more powerful plant is coffee. Everyone is aware of the stimulating effects of drinking too much coffee. It is important to monitor how much of that herb you drink each day because drinking too many cups will lead you to overdose on the plant. If you drink too much coffee each day, you will feel the effect in your body and you may experience long-term consequences of drinking too much. Imagine if you drank several cups of a strong diuretic tea each day: that would *definitely* have an effect on the body. Coffee is a great plant but should be used in moderation.

Know what's in your herbal tea blend

On the other hand, I have encountered plenty of people who think that herbs are so benign that they have no effect on the body at all. Herbal teas taste good, so people just drink them like beverages. But the plants in an herbal tea blend have an impact on the body, especially if the person is drinking a large quantity of tea. This was made clear to me by several people who work at healing centers that feature alternative-type therapies. In two places in particular, a signature herbal tea was served that had been created especially for their practice by a local herbalist.

Both "signature teas" contain plants that are nervines—that is, plants that calm and relax the nervous system. Because the teas were freely available and made in big batches every morning, the practitioners and clients helped themselves all day long. My friend, a Reiki practitioner, started noticing that she felt an increased lack of energy; some of her clients at the center reported such feelings, too. When I asked how much herbal tea she was drinking at work, she realized that she probably had been drinking three or more cups throughout the course of the day.

When I showed her the list of herbal plants in that "harmless" herbal tea she was drinking on a regular basis, she realized that her lack of energy could be attributed to the quantity of tea she was consuming and to the nervine herbs that the tea contained. She didn't need to be sedated: rather, she needed energy.

I find that the dosages in the chart below have worked well for me during the years I have worked with people. Of course, I modify my suggestions depending on the herbal plant, preparation, and weight and sensitivity of the person.

What is important is that you figure out what works for you and your family.

Take a Break

Herbs are used to correct body imbalances and to supplement the diet. Once we are better we stop taking the herbs. Herbs are not like drugs, they are not to be taken forever. Tonic herbs are taken for longer periods of time but it is recommended that you take a periodic break. For instance take 1 day off every week. Or take a week off every 4 weeks. People tend to do this naturally.

DOSAGE CHART FOR ADULTS

For acute imbalances:

Infusions: 3-4 cups daily. 1 tsp. – 1 Tbsp. dried herb to 1 cup water. Let steep for 20 minutes or more.

Decoctions: 2-3 cups daily. 1 tsp. dried herb to 1 cup water.

Capsules: 1-2 "00" capsules, three times daily.

Tinctures: ¼ tsp. - ½ tsp. Three times daily. Tinctures are the standard 1:5 ratio.

Syrups: 1-3 Tbsp. daily.

For chronic imbalances:

Infusions: 2-3 cups daily. 1 tsp. – 1 Tbsp. dried herb to 1 cup water. Let steep as above.

Decoctions: 1-2 cups daily.

Capsules: 1-2 "00" capsules, two to three times daily.

Tinctures: ¼ tsp. – ½ tsp. Two to three times daily.

Syrups: 1-2 Tbsp. daily.

For nutritional doses:

Infusions: 1 cup daily. 1 tsp. – 1 Tbsp. dried herb to 1 cup water. Let steep as above.

Decoction: 1 cup daily

Capsules: 1-2 "00" daily

Tinctures: ¼ - ½ tsp. daily

Syrups: 1 Tbsp. daily

DOSAGE CHART FOR CHILDREN

Determine the weight of the child. If the child is half the weight of an adult (which is considered to be 150 lbs.) use half the dosage for adults. Babies use much less.

Dosage chart for children:

Infusions: ¼ - ½ cups daily. 1 tsp. – 1 Tbsp. dried herb to 1 cup water. Let steep for 20 minutes or more.

Decoctions: ¼ - ½ cups daily.
1 tsp. dried herb to 1 cup water.

Capsules: 1 "0" capsule, three times daily.

Tinctures: 3 to 10 drops. Three times daily.
Tinctures are the standard 1:5 ratio.

Syrups: 1-3 tsp. daily.

Rules that have been established by the medical community for children:

Young's Rule:
Add 12 to the child's age. Divide the child's age by this total.

Example: Dosage for a 4-year-old: 4 divided by 16 = .25, or ¼ of adult dosage.

Cowling's Rule:
Divide the number of a child's next birthday by 24.

Example: Dosage for a child who is 3, turning 4 years old: 4 divided by 24 = .16 or ¹⁄₁₆ of the adult dosage.

Quick Conversion Chart

(Many herbal books are from Europe and use the metric system.)

1 teaspoon = 5 milliliters

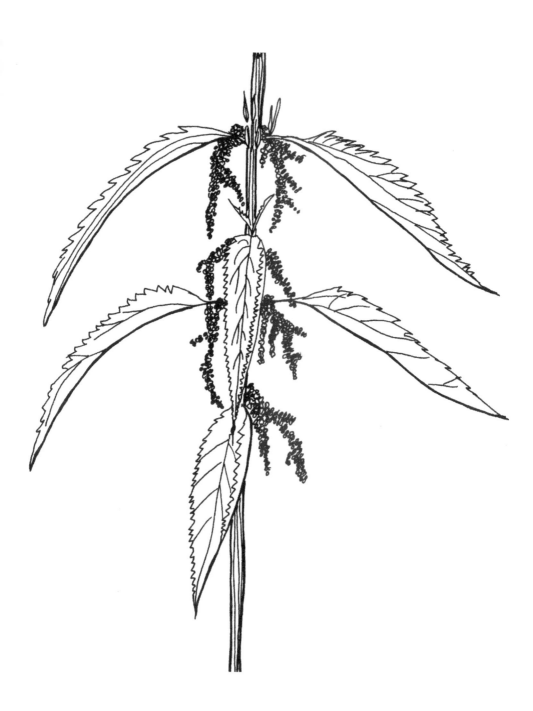

Chapter 6:

COLD OR FLU
OR ALLERGY

In my experience there is a difference between a cold and the flu. Although both colds and the flu can be viral, flu symptoms are different than cold symptoms.

The flu seems to affect the whole body. Its symptoms can include headache, aches and pains all over (especially in the bones), low to high fever, sore throat, a complete lack of energy, a strong need to sleep, lack of focus, and usually no appetite.

Cold symptoms can include sinus problems, earaches, coughing, sore throat, drippy nose, lack of energy, and stomach aches. Although these symptoms are annoying, they are not as physically debilitating as those experienced due to a bad case of the flu. In one way this is too bad because people think that they can just power through their daily routines and do not need to take the time to take extra care of themselves. Then they get much worse and have to slow down (or perhaps even come to a complete halt) because they have allowed themselves to become very sick.

Allergies

Allergy symptoms mimic cold symptoms more than flu symptoms. Allergies are caused by the substances that the body has decided it doesn't like, causing the respiratory system to overreact.

Sinus irritation, coughing, itchy and watery eyes, and sneezing are some allergy symptoms. In many cases, respiratory symptoms can lead to an infection and the person ends up with a cold. The respiratory herbs are very helpful in these cases.

A client of mine has seasonal allergies: they rear their ugly head during the fall season. She cleans her sinuses every night in fall with Sinus Steam and uses the Throat and Chest Remedy for the congestion in her lungs. Her allergies would turn into severe respiratory symptoms until she discovered that the herbs worked well; now, she takes them immediately if her allergies symptoms occur.

Flu Herbs

The herbal plants that treat colds and the flu are different as well. Traditionally, herbs that treat the flu cause a diaphoretic action which opens up the pores of the skin, helping the body to eliminate unwanted toxins. These herbal plants help the body relax, rest, sleep and ease the pain of the flu. Today people consider the action of a fever, which elevates the body temperature, as aiding the body's immune system in its effort to kill unwanted pathogens, so think twice about suppressing a fever with over-the-counter drugs. When my children were young it was customary to give children aspirin and acetaminophen (Tylenol) to reduce fevers.

At the time, fevers were considered bad and treatments sought to suppress their action in the body. There is a different approach to treating fevers in to-day's world. First of all, aspirin is considered to be too risky for children: Tylenol is toxic to the liver and can accumulate in the liver, putting young children (and adults) at risk. Caution is advised when using these over-the-counter drugs.

Catnip is an herb that is specific to children's imbalances. It helps a child rest and helps alleviate the fevers and pains that come with illness. The herbs in the Traditional Gypsy Flu Remedy have been used

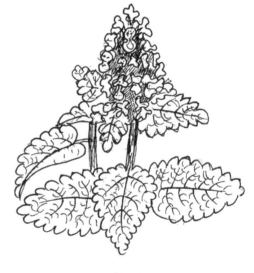

Catnip

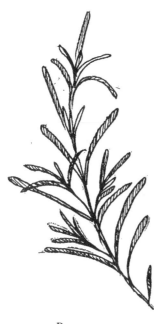

Rosemary

for centuries to treat flu symptoms. My addition of boneset, a plant that is indigenous to our country, makes the remedy a very effective infusion to take when suffering from the flu. Although boneset has a very bitter taste, people who have the flu that are aware of boneset's pain-relieving qualities just drink it down. Most of the time they are congested anyway and can't really taste it.

I have found that taste is entirely subjective. In my talks I have passed all kinds of different-tasting teas and tinctures around the classroom, and I am always amazed at the different reactions. Some people perceive certain herbs to be bitter while others find them to be sweet. Children, on the other hand, are so reluctant to drink anything unknown. Please refer to the **Children's Section** on how to prepare herbs for children.

In the case of colds I treat each individual symptom. My strongest herbal remedy for a bad cold is the Throat/Chest Remedy. I developed the recipe years ago when everybody had a weird version of a cold that seemed to lodge in the voice box or larynx. The combination of herbs works to move congestion out of the upper and lower respiratory systems. The remedy contains herbs that work as strong antimicrobials, herbs specific to the throat and lungs, and an expectorant that moves congestion out of the lungs by promoting coughing. It works particularly well for people who have a lingering cold or keep becoming re-infected and not getting better.

I recently received a phone call from a friend who was recovering from the flu. He had used my herbal flu and cold remedies very successfully in the past, but this time he called because he was concerned about new symptoms: he was coughing and unable to sleep.

Together, we figured out that before he had experienced these new symptoms, he had been suffering from a very bad case of the flu: then, his symptoms had included body aches and pains—plus he had just felt awful—but his respiratory system hadn't been involved. He wasn't stuffy, congested, or coughing, but he couldn't get out of bed for a week. I figured that because he had used all the herbal formulas in the past he would know

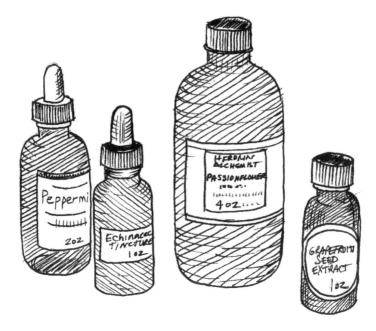

what to do. So I sent Gypsy Flu Remedy, the Throat/Chest Decoction, elderberries for a syrup, and the Garlic Honey Infusion. In his quest to get better fast, he made them in large quantities and took all the infusions, decoction and syrup at once.

He felt a lot better: his aches and pains were gone but now he had too much energy to sleep and coughing fits. He was concerned and justifiably so. All he needed to take was the Gypsy Flu Remedy but not the Throat/Chest Decoction because some of the herbs in that blend worked as expectorants. The expectorant herbs were making him cough when he didn't need to cough. The coughing was what prevented him from getting the sleep that he needed to recover. He called me up later and asked if he should have houseguests later in the week. I told him to meet them at the door with the herbal blends that he had just made—the Garlic Honey Infusion, Elderberry Syrup, and Echinacea Tincture—and everyone should be fine for the weekend.

Chapter 7

STAGES OF AN IMBALANCE

It is rare that we will come down with "something completely" with a set of terrible symptoms in 24 hours. Rather, we get sick in stages. It is more likely that your body will give warning signals all along. It pays to listen and learn to interpret your body's signals. My signs are a tickle in the back of my throat and a hoarse voice. Most of the times I do not feel "sick", just more tired than usual. This is the herbal window of opportunity.

I cannot emphasize enough how important it is to **slow down** *and* **heed these warnings.** *The time you spend taking care of yourself in the beginning of an imbalance will pay off in the end.*

Sleep

Remember the body repairs itself when it sleeps. Going to bed early or spending a day in bed is wonderful medicine. Don't wait until you are so sick that you cannot get out of bed. By then it is a long road to recovery.

Water

Drink water and lots of it. For me, one of the first signs of being ill is urinating too much, way more than I should be based on the amount of liquid I am consuming. My body's water ratio becomes imbalanced. Like most people, I struggle to drink a lot of water. I drink tea, herb tea, seltzer water, etc., but I

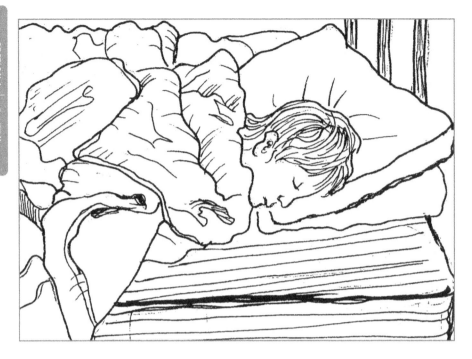

have to force myself to drink regular water. Keep a jug of water in the refrigerator because people like cold beverages. I like my water to be almost room temperature. Carry a water bottle. It is a wise idea to increase your water intake if you are not feeling up to par.

The Herbal Window of Opportunity

Using herbal medicine in the first stages of an illness is the most effective way of using herbs. There are several herbs that work as "preventatives". This means that they raise the body's defense mechanisms and target and eliminate the pathogens that are causing our symptoms.

Although you are not officially "sick", this is the time to start using herbs and herbal techniques to prevent a cold from taking hold. It has been my experience that people who have started to rest right away and take herbal medicines early do not get "sick". Several elderly people have told me that they consider this to be a miracle. They had resigned themselves to getting sick every winter; there was nothing you could do about it. I call Echinacea the "gateway herb" because once people experience its preventive actions they are interesting in exploring other herbs.

Herbal Preventatives when exposed to a sick environment

The other way herbs work as preventatives is when taken during periods of exposure to a sick environment. My friend is a barber and during the cold season she takes ¼ teaspoon of Echinacea Tincture every day so that she stays well. Although the herbal literature does not support this use of Echinacea, it is being used this way and is effective. During my twenty years of teaching, I have been asking students about their experiences with using Echinacea Tincture in this way and it does work for many people. I suggest using Elderberry Syrup in this manner as well.

My Favorite Herbal Preventatives

I have been interested in herbal plants that can be used as preventatives during the cold and flu season because knowing that you have the tools to prevent or avoid becoming sick gives people peace of mind. I like to use three herbal plants in this manner: echinacea, elderberry and garlic.

Echinacea

Echinacea works as an "immunostimulant". This means that it helps the body fight off an invading infection by raising the level of white blood cells in the blood. White blood cells are our immune system's weapon for fighting infection.

Echinacea needs to be taken in sufficient amounts, and I feel that the tincture preparation is the most effective. Echinacea has become a very popular flower garden plant with many differently-cultivated types of flowers, so if you make your own tincture make sure that you are using the medicinal species. Check out the **Plants Bio** section for growing information.

The literature (German Commission E) states that Echinacea should be

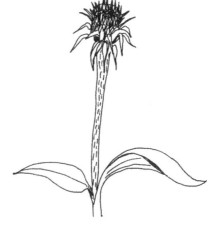

Echinacea Flower Bud

taken no longer than 2-3 weeks as it becomes ineffective. I have found that people do not take it that long because after a couple of days they are better. The one exception to this is people who are using it as a preventative because they work with the public. Usually they take it for several weeks and automatically take a break because the latest "cold/flu" outbreak has run its course. Ellingwood's *American Materia Medica* published in 1919 writes about the incredible uses of this plant for all types of infections.

Elderberry

I have been interested in plants that work as preventatives that you can take every day—herbs that work as tonics that can prevent one from becoming sick. Echinacea has always carried a warning about not taking it every day for long periods of time. So as a mother and an herbalist I was interested in a preventative herbal preparation that people would gladly take every day and I found it: Elderberry Syrup. The syrup is easy to make from dried elderberries. Elder bushes grow all over our area and it is easy to harvest the ripe berries in late summer (unless you are competing with the birds, who love the berries, too, and will pluck the ripe berries before you notice they are ripe). People love the taste of the syrup. Children will happily take their spoonful of delicious syrup every morning.

Garlic

Raw garlic is the best "antibiotic" in the plant kingdom. In a petri dish, everything will stay away from it. It is a very powerful antimicrobial which means it is anti-viral, anti-bacterial, and anti-fungal. I use fresh raw garlic from local farmers. At the end of the summer I stock up on the freshest local garlic and prepare it many ways (mostly, I use it in cooking). For medicinal recipes, I used to mince raw cloves and put it into capsules for my children. Nowadays, I make a honey infusion which is my favorite herbal preventative or I just spread the raw chopped garlic on bread.

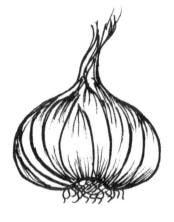

Garlic

Several years ago it seemed that I was surrounded by sickly twenty-year-olds. They were at work and in my house. They kept spreading their illnesses around and getting re-infected and, of course, were not taking care of themselves. So I made two huge batches of Garlic Honey Infusion and insisted that they all take a teaspoon every day until they got better. It worked. I also learned that not everyone can tolerate the strong stuff and that you can take it with a carrier cracker or piece of bread to help it go down.

Recovery Phase

When we turn a corner and start feeling better, it is important to still take the healing herbs and rest as we start to return to our daily routines (without just jumping back into it). One of the problems I have seen continuously is that people do not take the time to recover. They start to feel better and think that they are better. They are not. It takes time. The danger is that they don't recover properly and are vulnerable to catching another cold or flu very quickly. Or they never really get over the original cold or flu in the first place. It keeps flaring up. They never feel well for the whole winter season. A lack of energy and an inability to "feel normal" are big complaints. I suggest that if you still have symptoms or one symptom such as a cough that doesn't seem to go away, start using the appropriate herbs again for that problem and rest. I know the feeling of being sick and being tired of being sick.

Years ago I had a respiratory illness that I couldn't seem to shake. It kept coming back or it never went away. Although I had been to the doctor many times so that they could check my lungs, I couldn't seem to get over my "bug". I was taking herbal remedies so my symptoms were not as severe as they would have been under normal circumstances, but my symptoms were lingering on and on.

The doctors did not prescribe any drugs except the usual over-the-counter drugs. (At the time I remember being amazed by how limited the selection of medicines were in drugstores. I couldn't find any plant-based medicines at all.) I felt that I needed something more. Finally, I took a mild antibiotic that my grandson hadn't used and it was what I needed to get over the hump.

Although this book is about using plants as medicines, remember that there is a place for all types of medicines that are available to us.

The Role of Herbs in the Recovery Phase

There are several different categories of herbs that help us feel better and soothe the recovery phase.

- 🌿 Stimulant herbs that give the body energy
- 🌿 Stimulant herbs that boost the effectiveness of an herbal recipe
- 🌿 Tonic herbs that supply much-needed nutrition to give the body energy
- 🌿 Liver herbs that help the liver clear up unwanted toxins in the body (these herbs are sometimes referred to as blood purifiers
- 🌿 Adaptagen herbs for recuperating from an illness

It is time to start using nutritional herbs as well as plants that help the liver do its job when we start to feel better. My favorite herbal blend for recuperation contains the liver herb, burdock root, the adaptagen herb, Siberian ginseng, and the demulcent herb, licorice. It moves unwanted substances out of the body while providing some much-needed energy, and it tastes sweet because of the licorice.

Please refer to the **Immune System** and **Be Well** sections for further information on the herbal plants that help the body recover and be well.

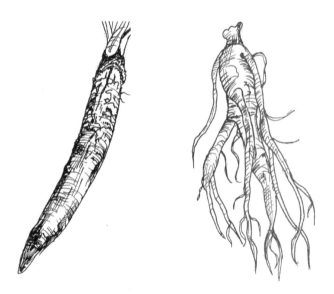

Burdock Root (left), Ginseng Root (right)

....

Chapter 8

CHILDRENS' SECTION

....

There is nothing more discouraging than preparing an herbal infusion or an herbal tincture only for your child to refuse to open his or her mouth; you just know that you aren't going to win the battle of getting him or her to take the herbal preparation you've lovingly made. All of your hard work turns out to be for nothing.

In my early days of using herbs I would make an infusion of the "correct" herb that I knew would help my children get better. I remember making an infusion of boneset, a traditional herb that helps the body move through a bout of flu. I have even seen it mentioned in a children's nursery rhyme in one of my mother's childhood books. It was the right herb for the job, but I had never tasted boneset by itself. I had used it in blends but never alone. I knew it tasted bitter, but when I tasted it on the day before I planned to give it to my son I realized that no matter how much honey I put into the cup there was no way he would drink it. It was way too bitter for his taste buds. So I put the infusion into a hot bath instead, where it calmed him down and helped alleviate the uncomfortable feeling of the flu.

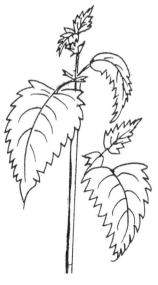

Now I use Catnip for my grandchildrens' baths. Catnip has a special affinity with children.

Catnip

Make it taste good or taste acceptable.

Herbal infusions can be sweetened with honey, maple syrup, rice syrup, fruit juice, stevia, or my favorite Elderberry syrup to make them taste good. I used to use grape juice to disguise a lot of weird tastes and *I* thought that it worked great (but maybe I should ask my kids how well it worked…).

Now, I use Elderberry Syrup as a sweetener. I make it in batches in the winter season. It is my go-to herbal preparation for disguising the tastes of other infusions, decoctions and tinctures. Alcohol tinctures do not taste very good to children: besides the alcohol taste, many of the herbs that are used for illnesses taste bitter. I have found that everyone loves the taste of Elderberry Syrup. Making the syrup takes some time but once you go through the preparation process you will have an herbal blend that can be used for months. Syrups work so well for children because they taste good and the dosages are small.

Hibiscus, fennel seed, licorice root, peppermint, spearmint, lemon balm and cinnamon can be added to an herbal mixture for flavor. Experiment with different flavors.

Remember adults who are just little children in larger bodies.

Herbal preparations are no good if nobody will take them and adults will gladly take an herbal preparation if it tastes good.

Serve it cold or frozen.

I didn't have much luck serving my small children warm tea. They didn't like any warm beverages. Only when my son grew older would he ask for a hot cup of peppermint tea when he was sick. Peppermint helped him and he would drink it down. Every child is different so see if your child likes warm tea. I hear from so many parents nowadays that their children love to drink warm tea.

Since my children didn't like warm beverages, I decided to serve their herbal infusions cold or frozen. I would combine herbal infusions or decoctions with grape juice or fruit juice and put the mixture into popsicle molds purchased from the store. I sometimes added Echinacea Tincture directly to the popsicle mixture before I froze it. This method worked so well for my son (who was plagued with ear infections) that the minute I saw him coming down with anything I made some herbal popsicles.

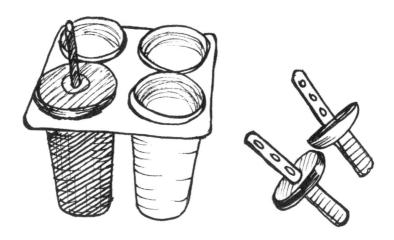

Label your creations.

I used to make quantities of a special nutritional tea for my adolescent daughter. I stored it in ½ gallon canning jars in the refrigerator and she'd just drink her herbal blend right out of the refrigerator. I will never forget the time she gulped down some cold tea from the refrigerator without looking at the label. She drank half of a quart jar and then looked at me with a panicked look on her face. She said: "What did I drink? It doesn't taste like my tea." I told her that she had just consumed a wonderful liver formula whose taste left something to be desired (at the time I was teaching about herbs for the digestive system). So label your creations: you never know who is visiting your refrigerator.

Use a Medicinal Dropper.

I have all sizes of glass droppers at my house from herbal tincture bottles. I found that my little grandson wouldn't drink the herbal blend I made him from a cup but would let me squirt the herbal blend into his mouth from a big dropper. Now he takes great delight in sucking up the herbal mixture by

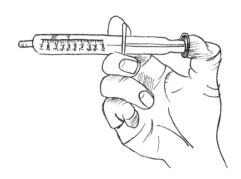

himself with a big plastic medicinal dropper; he squirts it into his mouth by himself. I just put his dosage of the herbal mixture into a cup and let him "do it himself". Drugstores carry all sizes of plastic medicinal droppers for use in dispensing children's drugs such as Motrin or Tylenol.

It is very important to dispense the correct dosage when using these drugs for children. Studies found that parents were having issues with dosages when dispensing drugs using small cups. Medicinal droppers were found to be easier to use to determine the correct dosage to give to children. The same holds true for dispensing herbal preparations. I suggest putting the desired measurements on the plastic droppers with a sharpie markers because many of the droppers use hard-to-read metric measurements. As you can see by the dosage charts, small children require small dosages of herbs. Use your measuring spoons and water to determine a teaspoon or tablespoon, mark them for future use and when it comes time to dispense an herbal preparation you'll be ready.

Medicinal Droppers also work great for dispensing herbal preparations to animals.

Use an Herbal Bath Preparation

Children love baths. Putting an herbal infusion into their bathwater is a method to use herbs for children. I gave my children yarrow baths every day when they were sick. Because of the diaphoretic actions of yarrow, I felt that it helped move the illness through their body quicker. After their yarrow baths I would wrap them up in blankets to sweat the illness out. This works great for adults, too, and if you don't feel like taking a bath just use a foot bath. I notice that people do not take baths anymore and in many cases do not have a bathtub in their bathrooms—just a shower stall.

Use an Herbal Smoothie Preparation

My daughter makes "green drinks" for her young children. She mixes a nutritional herbal powder with yogurt and banana and blends it with a handheld blender. She also adds a lemon-flavored cod liver oil. The drinks are delicious and the kids ask for them.

Use straws or sippy cups.

My daughter uses sippy cups for green drinks for her toddler. She made the top wider by cutting it down. It works well for the thick drink and keeps the mess to a minimum. She also uses cups with built-in straws in the lids.

Make a special bottle labeled with their name.

I put a small amount of elderberry syrup along with several drops of echinacea tincture in a small dropper bottle with my grandkids' names on it: they know that it's special "medicine" just for them. I let them squirt the mixture into their mouths by themselves. This is an effective way to get them to take their herbs.

Use capsules for teenagers.

Gelatins capsules come in various sizes. I use the '0' size for young adults because they are smaller. Teenagers seem to be more compliant when it comes to taking capsules and pills as opposed to other preparations. This is the same for many adults.

My favorite herbs for children are catnip, chamomile, fennel seed, spearmint, peppermint, and elderberries.

Glycerin Tinctures

Glycerin is a byproduct of the alcohol industry and it tastes very sweet. These tinctures use glycerin instead of alcohol as a base or menstrum. Glycerin tinctures are not as strong as alcohol-based tinctures and are uniquely suited for children. I did not use Glycerin Tinctures for my kids because they really didn't exist at that time: they were harder to make and their shelf life is much shorter than that of alcohol-based tinctures. This preparation has become very popular with parents because the kids love the sweet taste (though not all glycerin tinctures taste good, as I discovered when I broke down and bought a combination of Echinacea and goldenseal glycerin tincture for my four-year-old grandson: he absolutely refused to take any of my regular herbal preparations and needed help with his sinus cold). Oddly enough, it tasted pretty strange, I do not think anything can disguise the bitter taste of goldenseal. Most glycerin tinctures taste very good and if you have a fussy kid perhaps glycerin tinctures are the way to go.

Put herbal preparations out of reach of young children

*I advise making sure that all of your tinctures bottles and herbal preparations are kept where a small child **cannot** reach them.* Glycerin tinctures taste like candy and a small child will form an association between tincture bottles and good tastes. Parents are lulled into a false sense of security these days because of childproof caps on medicine bottles. I had a young son and now two grandsons and they manage to get into areas of the kitchen that you would never expect them to reach. As far as I know there are no childproof caps on any tincture bottles. This advice is for all herbal preparations. When my grandson was eighteen months old he ate a half-bottle of homeopathic pills for teething. He was fine—but not without a lot of worry from his parents.

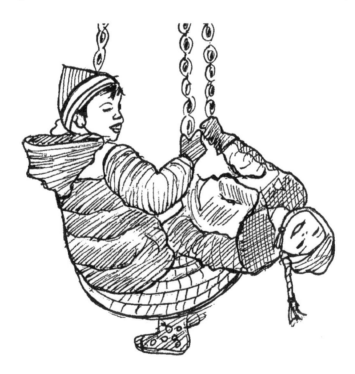

··

Chapter 9

LANGUAGE OF HERBALISM

··

In order to better understand how herbs work in the body, we need to use the centuries-old language of herbalism. The words describe the actions of the herbal plants in the body. For instance, antimicrobial herbs work by destroying or helping the body resist pathogenic microorganisms. They are anti-viral, anti-bacterial and anti-fungal because they work to eliminate these infections from the body.

Currently our medical system does not use the following terms because they have a different approach to understanding how the body works and a different set of tools they are trained to use (pharmaceutical drugs and surgery).

Imbalances

Herbalists use the word "imbalance" to describe an illness. There are all types of imbalances ranging from weak to strong. This book addresses the acute imbalances that occur when the body succumbs to the cold and flu.

Tonics

The term "tonic" is not used in our current medical language, though it is a very commonly-used term in herbalism to describe the actions of most herbs. I consider the tonic herbs to symbolize the way in which herbal actions are most effective in the body. Most herbs work like highly nutritious food in the body. Herbal plants are loaded with nutrients and they work by supplying the needed nutrition that the body needs especially during times of sickness.

Tonic herbs are integral to helping the body get better. Pharmaceuticals drugs do not work as tonics.

"Specifics"

Herbal plants have an affinity for different body systems and the imbalances that can happen within a particular body system. Plants that work to alleviate an imbalance of a particular body system or symptom are called "specifics". Sage tea (yes, that sage plant, the turkey sage) is specific for sore throats. It works well as a gargle and as a tea. It also makes a tasty tea or infusion.

"Specifics" for Cold and Flu Symptoms

Herbal plants have been used for centuries to treat colds and the flu. The combination of elder flower, peppermint, yarrow, and catnip is a traditional gypsy remedy for colds and flu that dates back hundreds of years. This combination helps the digestive, nervous and respiratory systems overcome the symptoms that characterize the winter flu. The old Herbals (books that were written centuries ago about medicinal plants) mention the same plants time and time again as remedies for certain symptoms. These same plants are just as effective today. Peppermint stills works to alleviate digestive imbalances. Catnip (as a tea or an infusion) is the best herb for children.

Action Herbs for Colds and the Flu

During a time of illness or imbalance (an herbalist's term for sickness) plants work to stimulate the immune system by supporting its ability to function properly. Plants help the immune system to resist incoming infections and soothe the mucous membranes of the sinuses, lungs, and the digestive system. They help the nervous system calm down, allowing the body to get the rest it needs. The following terms describe the actions of the herbal plants that are used to treat imbalances. The plants that are used the most when sick fall into four categories: anti-microbial, diaphoretics, demulcents and expectorants. These plants have a front row seat in moving the sickness out of the body and soothing the body systems so that one feels better.

Antimicrobial

Plants work as "antimicrobials". Because many plants and plant preparations such as essential oils contain substances that are anti-bacterial, anti-viral and anti-fungal, they are effective in treating both colds and flu. Antibiotics are only anti-bacterial, not anti-viral: therefore, they do not work well when treating viral infections such as the flu. Many culinary herbs such as thyme, garlic and rosemary are filled with volatile oils that are antimicrobial.

Traditionally, these herbs were used to flavor as well as protect the people who consumed these foods. Cooking with these culinary herbs that work medicinally helps our bodies stay healthy throughout the winter season.

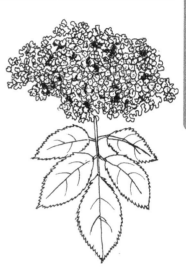

Elder Flower

Antimicrobial herbs:

Flower: Calendula, Elder, Yarrow

Leaf: Echinacea, Eucalyptus

Root: Elecampane, Goldenseal, Licorice, Oregon Grape, Osha, Marshmallow

Bulb: Garlic

Bark: Pau D'Arco

Fruit: Cayenne, Elder

Extracts: Grapefruit Seed Extract, Oregano Oil

Resin: Myrrh

Bud: Clove

51

Diaphoretic Herbs

Sometimes when we are ill, the elimination organs are not working as well as they should and certain herbal plants will help the body release its waste products through the skin by opening the pores and promoting the action of sweating. The body releases toxins in the system through the skin, taking the burden off of the kidneys and the lungs. These herbs, called diaphoretics, help hasten the healing process. This is the same concept behind sauna baths and American Indian sweat lodges.

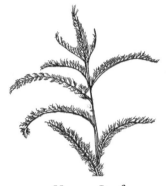

Yarrow Leaf

Boneset, yarrow and elder flower have been used this way for centuries to treat influenza. I use these herbs externally in herbal baths as well as internally. Bathing with diaphoretic herbs is a very effective form of preparation, especially for children. After using diaphoretic herbs in the bath it is important to cover up the whole body with blankets to continue the sweating process. The pores are open so it is important to not let the body get chilled. Diaphoretic plants are also used to treat chills that accompany colds and the flu. Diaphoretics are not to be used with high fevers.

I used yarrow herbal baths extensively with my children as well as myself. My children were not prone to high fevers (in fact, they usually had mild fevers with their illnesses). So I got in the habit of preparing yarrow baths each day during their illness. I would then wrap them up in blankets after their baths and hope that they would fall asleep.

Today people look at the action of a fever with its elevated body temperature as aiding the body immune system in killing off unwanted pathogens.

Diaphoretic Herbs:

Leaf/Flowers: Boneset, Yarrow, Elder Blossoms

Root: Ginger

Use: fevers, colds

Demulcent Herbs

Demulcent herbs are rich in mucilage, a constituent of plants that when mixed with water creates a thick liquid. Some herbs are very rich in mucilage such as marshmallow root and slippery elm bark. The resulting tea or decoction helps protect and soothe the mucous membranes in the sinuses, throat, lungs, and the gastrointestinal tract that might be irritated or inflamed. These plants work well as decoctions and infusions by themselves, or demulcents can be added to other recipes to temper stronger action herbs. This category of plants is so important because they are very healing to the body especially when one is ill. Marshmallow Root is my go-to herb when dealing with colds and the flu because usually the respiratory system is involved. I use it in so many recipes for the lungs and sinuses.

Demulcent herbs:

Leaf: Oats

Bark: Slippery Elm Bark

Roots: Marshmallow Root, Licorice

Use: sinus, throat, lungs, stomach conditions

Expectorant

"Expectorant" is a misunderstood term. Originally, it described a plant that loosens mucous secretions from the lungs and promotes coughing as a way to eliminate the mucous from the lungs. Sometimes the person has a dry irritating cough that an expectorant would only make worse. There is a time and place for promoting coughing.

Expectorants produce a range of actions, from mild to very strong: one of my friends learned this the hard way by taking a Chinese herbal formula without knowing what it did. She took it because her friend said it worked for her cold. It was a strong expectorant formula and promoted coughing to clear the lungs. My friend did not have that type of cold and ended up coughing all day and all night long before she called me to find out what was the problem.

I have seen this word on many cough syrup bottles that do not actually contain any expectorant herbs. I remember a particular herbal cough syrup that was being advertised as an expectorant cough syrup that was being promoted as "quieting" the cough. Quieting the cough would be the job of antitussive herbs.

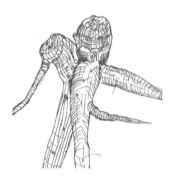

Elecampane Root

Expectorant herbs:

Leaf: Coltsfoot, Hyssop, Horehound, Lomatium, Plantain

Roots: Elecampane, Licorice,

Use: Congestion in respiratory system

Antitussive

Antitussive refers to the action of quieting the coughing reflex. It is very helpful for an annoying cough that is keeping a child from sleeping. It is not always wise to sedate every cough, as coughing can be very productive in the case of certain respiratory illnesses. The coughing reflex helps clear the mucous from the lungs.

Antitussive herbs:

Leaf: Mullein

Root: Wild Cherry Bark

Use: Sedate a cough

Catarrh

Catarrh refers to excessive secretion of the mucous membranes, a symptom of illness or allergies. A runny nose is one of the most complained about symptoms of a cold or allergy.

Anticatarrh

Anticatarrh refers to the preventing and drying up of excessive mucous in the body.

Anticatarrh herbs:

Leaf/Flower: Boneset, Cayenne, Elder, Elecampane, Hyssop, Mullein, Peppermint, Sage, Yarrow

Root: Goldenseal

Use: runny nose, dripping sinus

Antispasmodic

Antispasmodic herbs help soothe muscle tissue to prevent cramping.

Antispasmodic herbs:

Leaf: Peppermint, Motherwort, Skullcap,

Root: Crampbark, Valerian

Use: soothes intestinal cramping, calms the body

Adaptagens

....

"Adaptagen" is a relatively new term in the herbal world. It refers to an herb that helps the body adapt to stress. It works to balance the activity of the nervous, hormonal and immune systems.

Adaptagen herbs:

Leaf: Green Tea, Tulsi

Root: Astragalus, Ginseng (Panax and American), Siberian Ginseng (Eleutheroccus), Rhodiola

Mushroom: Reishi, Fungi Kingdom

Use: Physical wellbeing. To help cope with stressful situations.

Analgesic

....

An analgesic is an herb that relieves pain.

Analgesic herbs:

Leaf: Chamomile, Meadowsweet, Skullcap

Root: Ginger, Kava, Valerian

Bark: Willow Bark

Fruit: Cayenne

External analgesic herbs:

Arnica, St. John's Wort

Use: Helps aches and pain, sunburn, bruising.

Anti-inflammatory

Anti-inflammatories soothe inflammations and reduces the inflammation of the body tissues.

Anti-inflammatory herbs:

Leaf/Flower: Calendula, Chamomile, Meadowsweet, Yarrow, Plantain

Root: Turmeric, Ginger, Licorice

Bark: Willow Bark

External anti-inflammatory:

Oil: Arnica, St. John's Wort, Calendula

Poultice: Turmeric, Ginger

Use: inflammation

Anti-histamine

Anti-histamines block the action of the chemical "histamine" which the body produces as an allergic response.

Anti-histamine herbs:

Leaf: Nettle

Seed: Milk Thistle

Root: Burdock Root, Dandelion Root

Use: Control the allergic response

Carminatives

Carminative plants are rich in volatile oils that stimulate the digestive system to do its job. They relax the stomach and gastrointestinal tract.

Carminative herbs:

Leaf/Flower: Chamomile, Peppermint, Sage, Thyme

Root: Cinnamon, Ginger

Seed: Dill, Fennel, Anise

Fruit: Papaya

Use: Digestive conditions such as a stomach cramps, colic, indigestion

Inhalant

"Inhalant" refers to the inhalation of medicated air for therapeutic purposes. I grew up with Vick's VapoRub rubbed on the chest and under the nose to clear congestion caused by a cold or flu. It contains the essential oils of camphor, eucalyptus, and menthol in a salve preparation. My Sinus Steam recipe contains the plants that are high in volatile oils such as rosemary and thyme (which is why it works so well).

Inhalant herbs:

Leaf/Flower: Thyme, Calendula, Marshmallow, Sage, Rosemary

Essential Oil Preparations

Use: Clear the congestion of sinuses and lungs.

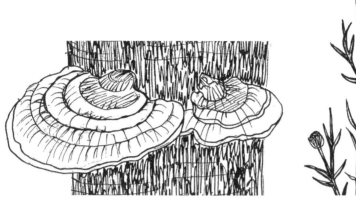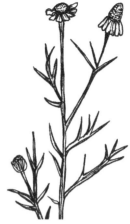

Reishi (left), Chamomile leaves and flowers (right)

Immunostimulant

Immunostimulants stimulate the functioning of the immune system. Echinacea promotes the production of white blood cells which work to combat acute infections in the body. Astragalus works as a tonic, building up the health of the immune system over a period of time, so it should be used after the body has recovered from an illness.

Immunostimulant herbs:

Leaf/Flower: Echinacea, Elder Blossoms

Root: Echinacea, Ginsengs, Licorice, Astragalus

Bark: Pau D'Arco

Bulb: Garlic

Mushroom: Reishi

Use: For acute infections such as a cold and as tonic
herb to prevent illness.

Laxative

Laxatives stimulate bowel movements. They help the digestive system do its job of elimination. There are two basic laxative herbs. The first category includes plants that contain fiber such as fruit, vegetables and seeds such as rhubarb or flax seeds. These work in the system as "bulk laxatives". They help move the waste matter down the GI tract. The second category of herbs includes plants that stimulate the peristalsis action of the muscles in the GI tract. Senna is a popular herb that causes cramping associated with the muscular action of the GI tract which in turn helps the digestive system work.

Laxative herbs:

Leaf: Senna, Cascara Sagrada

Root: Rhubarb, Dandelion Root, Yellow Dock, Licorice

Seed: Flaxseed, Psyllium

Preventatives

Preventatives strengthen and nourish specific organs as well as the whole body.

Preventative herbs:

Leaf/Flower: Echinacea, Elder, Yarrow

Berry: Elderberry

Root: Echinacea

Bulb: Garlic

Use: Take at first sign of imbalance to prevent illness

Pulmonary and Pectorals

Pulmonaries and pectorals refer to plants that are lung tonics. They are used to help correct lung imbalances and to strengthen the actions of the respiratory system.

Pulmonary herbs:

Leaf: Mullein, Thyme, Plantain, Hyssop, Coltsfoot

Root: Elecampane, Licorice, Marshmallow Root

Bark: Slippery Elm

Use: cough, lung congestion

Sedative or Nervine

Nervines affect the actions of the nervous system. The term usually refers to herbs that calm and sedate the nervous system rather than herbs like coffee that stimulate the nervous system. Sedative herbs reduce stress and calm the nervous system.

Sedating herbs:

Leaf/Flower: Catnip, Lavender, Passionflower, Skullcap

Root: Valerian

Use: Calming the body and promoting sleep during times of imbalances.

Stimulant

Stimulants are herbs that quicken the body's natural response; they increase the actions of the organ systems and the whole body's metabolism. Caffeine is the stimulating substance that is found in coffee. It stimulates our metabolism to work faster without the benefit of eating nutritious food. Cayenne and ginger are stimulating herbs that are used during an illness to hasten the body's metabolism, helping it to move the cold or flu through its process quicker.

Stimulating herbs:

Leaf: Coffee, Black Tea, Green Tea, Peppermint,
Yerba Matte, Rosemary

Root: Ginger

Fruit: Cayenne

Chapter 10

THE ROLE OF THE RESPIRATORY SYSTEM

The respiratory system's primary function is to supply oxygen to the body and dispose of the byproduct of respiration, carbon dioxide. It is divided into two regions: upper and lower. The upper respiratory system consists of the sinus cavities, nose, and throat (larynx and pharynx), and the lower respiratory system consists of the lungs. The lungs do the work of respiration, or the exchange of gases, and the sinuses, nose and throat help clean, warm, and purify the air before it enters the lungs.

Actions of the Herbs for the Respiratory System

Anti-microbial herbs that combat infection in the respiratory system (especially important to fight sinus infections)

Leaf/Flowers: Thyme, Calendula, Elder Blossoms, Elderberries, Echinacea

Root: Echinacea, Goldenseal, Oregon Grape, Licorice

Bulb: Garlic

Resin: Myrrh

Extract: Grapefruit Seed Extract, Olive Leaf Extract

Fruit: Cayenne

Anti-catarrh herbs help decrease catarrh or mucous from the sinuses and lungs

Leaf/Flower: Goldenrod, Elder, Peppermint, Red Clover Blossoms, Mullein, Hyssop

Root: Goldenseal

Resin: Myrrh

Essential Oils of Lavender, Rosemary, Peppermint

Anti-histamines dry up histamines (reaction from allergic response)

Leaf: Nettles

Astringents reduce irritation and inflammation by creating a barrier against infections

Leaf: Sage, Yarrow, Plantain

Diaphoretics help the body cope with illness by promoting sweating

Leaf/Flower: Boneset, Elder Blossoms, Yarrow, Catnip

Demulcents soothe and protect mucous membranes

Root: Slippery Elm Bark, Marshmallow Root, Licorice

Antitussives sedate the coughing reflex

Bark: Wild Cherry Bark

Root: Valerian Root

External Therapies

Steam inhalation

Leaf/Flower: Marshmallow, Chamomile, Thyme, Calendula, Rosemary, Sage

Nasal Wash

Salt

Gargle

Leaf: Sage

Bath/Foot Bath

Leaf: Yarrow, Marshmallow, Oats, Calendula, Roses, Lavender, Chamomile, Catnip

Poultices

Onion

Ginger

Heating Pads

Placed on the parts of the body that are
affected such as the ears or chest.

Warm air Humidifier/Vaporizer

Essential oils of lavender or rosemary diluted with water in the
appropriate container of the machine. Do not add it to the water
because it will break down the plastic parts of the machine.

Things to watch out for in the Winter Season

Dry Heat
It is a long winter here and no matter what type of heating you have in
your home or office it creates a drying atmosphere which is hard on the
respiratory system.

Woodstoves
Woodstove heat is incredibly drying and irritating to the sinus and lungs.
Our winter season is long in the North Country which means those stoves
are being used from November into May. Besides causing dry air, a woodstove pulls an incredible amount of oxygen out of the existing air in the
house in order to function properly. Even if you have an outside air venting
source, it still sucks the oxygen out of the atmosphere.

I have come across many people who think that they have had a cold all
winter long but really are suffering from irritation from woodstove heat. It
produces similar symptoms to an infection such as a cough, headaches, and
post nasal drip (which irritates the throat).

Air Exchange
The house needs regular air exchange during the winter and spring months.
Open up the windows and get some oxygen-laden air in the house.

Go Outside

It is imperative to get outside not only for the sake of the sun but for the oxygen-rich air of the winter months.

Add Moisture to the Air

It is also important to add moisture to indoor air, especially if you are having respiratory problems. There are several methods to add moisture to the atmosphere of the house.

Warm air Humidifiers/Vaporizers

One important way to increase the humidity of indoor air is to run a warm air humidifier in your bedroom at night while sleeping. For some reason, the use of warm air humidifiers is discouraged by the medical establishment. Most of the humidifiers that have been on the market in the last twenty years are cold air humidifiers (which do not work), so people have abandoned the use of humidifiers in the sickroom all together.

I tried using many cold air types: they made a lot of noise and didn't increase the humidity at all. The concern is that the warm air humidifiers will increase bacteria in the air. When they are used properly and are cleaned on a regular basis, they are an invaluable asset for helping people breathe at night when congested. The humidifier machines break down into several parts which can cleaned by running them through the dishwasher or handwashing them.

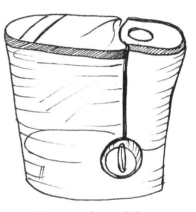

Warm air humidifier

I suggest taking the trouble of setting them up in the bedroom at the slightest suggestion of sinus difficulties.

So many parents use them in their children's' bedroom but not for their bedroom. Buy as many humidifiers as you have bedrooms. People in a family tend to get sick at the same time.

I run my humidifier all winter long and probably replace it every couple of years. It is totally worth the cost in terms of my respiratory health. I consider it invaluable when dealing with a sinus condition.

Most humidifiers have a cup that can be filled with essential oils. I suggest using a few drops of lavender or rosemary essential oils diluted in water for the medicine cup. A word of caution about using eucalyptus essential oil: it can be stimulating, so using it in a sickroom would not be helpful, especially for children.

Upper Respiratory System:
Sinuses, Ears, Nose, Voice Box, Throat

Sinuses

Sinuses help cleanse and condition the air that we breathe. Sinuses are the first line of defense against the seen and unseen mixtures of gases and toxins that is in our air. They consists of many large mucous-lined cavities in the head including special eye and ear cavities. They all produce secretions which drain down the nasal passages and into the throat cavity.

Sinus Problems

The sinuses can become irritated especially in the winter months simply from the lack of humidity in the air. They become infected and inflamed from allergic reactions to a variety of food allergies and irritating particles in the air: viruses, fungi and bacteria can contribute to sinus problems. Symptoms of sinus problems include excess mucous which results in a constant runny nose and headaches because of the swollen mucous membranes of the sinus cavities. It is advisable to start using strong herbal remedies right away to halt the spread of a sinus infection. Unlike many colds and flu, sinus problems take a long time to get better if left untreated. Treat early and often.

Herbs Specific for Sinuses

Leaf/Flower: Mullein, Thyme, Rosemary, Calendula, Hyssop, Peppermint, Echinacea, Golden Rod

Root: Goldenseal, Marshmallow, Horseradish, Ginger, Licorice, Osha

Bulb: Garlic

Resin: Myrrh

Infusions for Sinuses Imbalance

Leaf: Mullein, Goldenrod, Peppermint, Hyssop
Recipes: Sinus Clearing Remedy, Breathe Easy

Decoctions for Sinus Imbalance

Root: Marshmallow Root, Licorice, Ginger
Recipes: Throat Decoction, Children's Respiratory Blend

Powder/Capsules for Sinus Imbalance

Root: Goldenseal, Marshmallow
Recipe: Cold Cap/Yellow Pills

Syrups for Sinus Imbalance

Recipes: Elderberry, Ginger, Throat Health

Honey Infusions for Sinus Imbalance

Garlic/Honey Infusion

Food for Sinus Imbalance

Horseradish, Onions, Garlic

External Therapy for Sinus Imbalance
Caution: I don't recommend using essential oils for steam inhalations. Essential oils are extremely strong and very expensive. If you do want to use them, put several drops of essential oil in a teaspoon of carrier oil and then only use a couple of drops of the diluted oil. People complain of headaches and the drying out of their sinuses when using even one drop of essential oil in a steam inhalation. Fresh dried plants are brimming with volatile oils which are activated by rehydrating them with boiling water. The resulting steam is very effective but not so strong as to cause problems.

Steam Inhalation for Sinus Imbalance:

Leaf/Flower: Thyme, Rosemary, Marshmallow

Recipe: Sinus Steam Remedy

Baths/Foot Baths for Sinus Imbalance

Leaf: Yarrow

Recipe: Cleansing Bath, Traditional Gypsy Remedy

Nasal Wash for Sinus Imbalance

Neti Pot

Heating Pads

Place a warm pad over the forehead and eyes area

Warm air Humidifier/Vaporizers

Essential oils of Lavender or Rosemary

Nose

The nose is an organ of smell and warms, moisturizes and filters inhaled air as it passes into the respiratory system.

Runny Nose: The biggest complaint of colds, allergies, and flu is a runny nose. A clear or white discharge comes from colds or allergies. When the discharge changes color (yellow and green) there is an infection present.

Over-the-counter drugs like decongestants and antihistamines work to shrink mucus membranes and open nasal passages but they are very strong and many have a stimulating effect. They suppress the symptoms rather than work with the body to rid itself of the virus.

These herbal plants work to move the virus or imbalance out of the body. They thin out sticky and thick mucous, making it easier for mucous to drain. They have antimicrobial properties to combat infection.

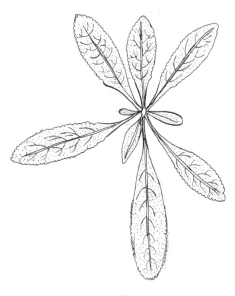

Mullein

Infusions for Runny Nose:

Leaf/Flower: Goldenrod, Elder, Calendula, Mullein, Yarrow, Catnip, Peppermint, Tulsi, Echinacea

Recipe: Sinus Clearing Remedy, Breathe Easy

Decoctions for Runny Nose:

Root: Elecampane, Marshmallow, Licorice, Ginger

Recipe: Throat Health, Children's Respiratory Blend

Powder/Capsule for Runny Noses:

Root: Goldenseal

Recipe: Cold Caps/Yellow Pills

Mouth

Cold Sores or Fever Blisters

Cold sores are caused by the herpes 1 virus which is related to the chicken pox virus. Once the nerve cells are infected they stay infected, and the virus stays dormant until it is activated by stress, a cold or other factors. Applying an anti-viral herb such as licorice in tincture-form directly onto the cold sore is extremely effective especially if it is used in the beginning stages of the eruption. Place a small amount of the tincture in a separate dropper bottle and apply to the cold sore as soon as you feel it happening. Keep applying all day long. Applying the licorice tincture (which tastes sweet) several times an hour in the beginning stages often eliminates the cold sores before they break through the skin.

I know many people who suffer from cold sores who make sure they have a supply of licorice tincture available all year round.

Lemon Balm has been found to be effective for the herpes virus and can be applied externally in a tincture or an ointment form.

The alcohol of these tinctures can irritate mucous membranes so an oil/cream/salve preparation would also be effective.

This information also applies to the herpes 2 virus which affects the genital area as well as shingles which is also a type of virus that affects the nerve endings of the skin.

External Therapies

Cold Sores (herpes 1 & 2 virus) and Shingles

Licorice Tincture applied directly to cold sore as soon as it feels like an eruption might occur. This works better than any other preparation.

Tinctures: Licorice, St. John's Wort, Lemon Balm

Oil preparations to be used externally

Oils: St. John's Wort, Lemon Balm, Lavender

Internal Therapies

Infusions for cold sores

Leaf/Flower: Calendula, Lemon Balm

Decoctions for cold sores

Root: Marshmallow, Licorice

Recipe: Cold Sore Blend

Tinctures for cold sores

Licorice, St. John's Wort, Lemon Balm, Echinacea

Throat

The throat is composed of the throat canal and the larynx or voice box. It is susceptible to all kinds of problems. Environmental factors such as smoke and dry heat can cause irritation in the throat which can lead to something more serious. Colds and the flu affect the throat in several places. Several years ago there was a virus that seemed to stay lodged in the larynx or voice box. I found that a combination of throat herbs and strong antimicrobial herbs worked well to alleviate that particular virus.

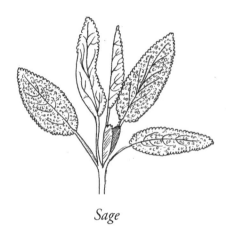

Sage

Tonsils are composed of lymph tissue which is at the back of the throat. Tonsils can become infected, causing a condition known as tonsillitis (which is more prevalent in children). In the recent past, it was believed that removing the tonsils would prevent illness from reoccurring. I still remember my

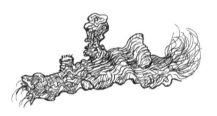

Osha Root

tonsil operation in the 1950s. Today the medical community views the tonsils as part of the immune system's response: they are the first line of defense against infection, localizing the infection before it gets further into the body.

Strep Throat is a bacterial infection. Strep Throat is treated with antibiotics. Its symptoms are similar to a viral infection so it is diagnosed by a throat culture.

Throat Congestion:

Infusion for Throat Congestion

Leaf: Sage, Peppermint
Recipe: Sinus Clearing Remedy

Decoction for Throat Congestion

Root: Marshmallow, Licorice, Osha
Bark: Slippery Elm
Recipe: Throat Health Recipe

Tinctures for Throat Congestion

Osha, Goldenseal, Echinacea, Sage, Thyme

Powder/Capsules for Throat Congestion

Cold Caps/Yellow Pills

External Therapies

Gargle for Throat Congestion

Sage Infusion
Cayenne Infusion

Sore Throat

Infusions for Sore Throat

Leaf: Sage, Peppermint, Chamomile, Mullein
Recipe: Sore Throat Remedy, Breathe Easy

Vinegar Extracts for Sore Throat

Apple Cider Vinegar/Honey Drink

Winter Root Vinegar in hot water

Lemon Drink for Sore Throat

Lemon/Honey Remedy with cayenne or garlic

Decoctions for Sore Throat

Root: Marshmallow, Licorice, Osha

Bark: Slippery Elm

Recipe: Throat Health, Children's Respiratory Blend

Tinctures for Sore Throat

Osha, Sage, Echinacea, Calendula, Thyme, Myrrh, Licorice

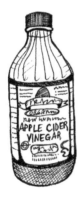
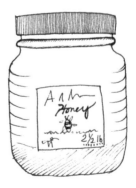

External Therapies

Gargle for Sore Throat

Sage Infusion, Calendula Infusion

Herbal Throat Spray

Echinacea Tincture, diluted

Licorice Tincture, diluted

Adult and Children's Throat Spray recipes

Additional

Warm Air Humidifier/Vaporizer

Post Nasal Drip

Post nasal drip becomes a problem when excess secretions from the sinuses drain down the back of the throat. The "drip" or drainage causes voice congestion and tickles the back of the throat causing an annoying cough. This coughing can be prominent at night, preventing a restful sleep. As excess secretions drain into the stomach, indigestion can occur. See "Herbs for Cough" below and review the **Digestion** section for more information.

Infusion for Post Nasal Drip

Leaf/Flower: Peppermint, Mullein, Sage, Chamomile, Hyssop

Seed: Fennel

Recipe: Post Nasal Drip, Breathe Easy, Sinus Clearing Remedy

Decoction for Post Nasal Drip

Root: Marshmallow, Licorice, Ginger

Bark: Slippery Elm

Recipe: Smooth Digestion

Syrup for Post Nasal Drip

Throat Health

Infusions for Post Nasal Drip Indigestion

Leaf: Peppermint, Chamomile, Spearmint

Seed: Fennel

Decoctions for Post Nasal Drip Indigestion

Root: Ginger

Seed: Fennel

Ears

My son's reoccurring earaches throughout childhood is the main reason I am an herbalist today. Earaches are the most common complaint of children. They can be very painful because the fluid that builds up in the middle ear can create quite a bit of pressure. Twenty-five years ago this condition (called "otitis media") was treated by an operation that inserted tiny ventilation tubes into the eardrum to help drain the fluid. Long term antibiotics (to be used all winter long) was the only other treatment.

After my small child underwent two ear operations, I told my ears, throat, and nose doctor that there must be a better way. I was completely frustrated. He started yelling at me for questioning the treatment options, saying that there was not another way—that the operations were the very latest options in scientific medicine. I never went back to him and did find a better way. I started studying in earnest the use of plants as medicines.

I found that treating my son with herbs helped halt or slow the progress of the cold or flu. I would watch for those "first signs" that he was catching something. Immediately, I would give him Echinacea tincture (I used an alcohol-based tincture, as glycerin tinctures were not available at that time) in a small amount of grape juice several times a day. That helped boost his immune system. He took yarrow herb baths every day. The diaphoretic herb helped move the toxins out of his system. After the bath I wrapped him up in blankets and put him to bed. I made sure he had lots of bedrest. I watched what he ate. I fed him soups and no sugary drinks or milk products.

I put chopped garlic in small capsules for him to swallow to work as an antibiotic. I made herbal popsicles which contained herbal infusions and decoctions flavored with grape juice. Sometimes I made herbal teas to alleviate his symptoms. He didn't like hot teas, but once in a while he would drink peppermint tea which helped to clear congestion.

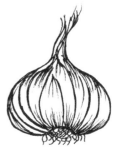

Garlic

I warmed up kosher salt in a cast iron pan until it was very warm and poured it into two tube socks to place on his ears for comfort and pain relief.

In the beginning, it seemed like he would get an earache immediately if he was getting sick, but I later found out that that wasn't the case. He was just very sensitive about his ears because of his history of ear problems.

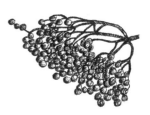

Elderberries

As I discovered which herbs and herbal preparations worked, I felt a sense of confidence that I had indeed found a better way.

Use preventative herbal remedies such as Elderberry Syrup during the winter season to strengthen the immune system.

Otoscopes are useful to check what is happening in the ear canal. They can be purchased at a health store. I found that food allergies can contribute to ear problems: for instance, excessive intake of dairy and fruit juices can contribute to congestion in the respiratory system.

Treat early and often.

See Children's Section for special preparations and dosages.

Herbs specific for ear imbalances

Infusions for Ear Imbalances:

Leaf: Peppermint, Elder Blossoms, Catnip, Mullein

Recipe: Breathe Easy, Traditional Gypsy Flu Remedy, Sinus Clearing Remedy

Decoctions for Ear Imbalances:

Root: Marshmallow, Licorice

Recipe: Children's Respiratory Remedy, Throat Health

Tinctures for Ear Imbalances:

Echinacea, Echinacea Glycerin, Goldenseal, Thyme, Yarrow

Honey Infusion for Ear Imbalances:

Garlic Honey

Syrups for Ear Imbalances:

Elderberry Syrup, Children's Respiratory Remedy, Throat/Chest Decoction

External Therapies

External Herbal Oil for Ear Imbalances

Mullein Flower or Garlic Oil

Bath/Foot Bath for Ear Imbalances:

Leaf: Yarrow, Catnip
Recipe: Cleansing Bath

Additional

Hot packs on ears

Warm Air Humidifier/Vaporizer

Eyes

Pink Eye or conjunctivitis is a bacterial or viral infection that is common in children. It is very contagious. The eyes are swollen and secrete a thick discharge which makes the eyelids stick together. Eye irritation is also a symptom of colds and the flu.

Besides using antimicrobial herbs internally, the best method to treat eyes is an herbal compress. Soak a small, clean cloth in a warm herbal infusion and place over the closed eyes for 5-10 minutes. Use the herbal compress to wipe the secretions from the eyes.

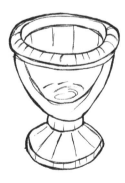

Eye cup

Infusions for Eye Imbalances:

Leaf/Flower: Catnip, Calendula

Recipe: Eye Imbalance, Breathe Easy, Children's Respiratory Blend

Decoctions for Eye Imbalances

Root: Marshmallow, Licorice

Berry: Elder

Syrups for Eye Imbalances

Elderberry Syrup, Children's Respiratory Blend

Tinctures for Eye Imbalances

Echinacea, Goldenseal

External Therapies

Compress for Eye Imbalances

Leaf/Flower: Calendula, Chickweed

Recipe: Sinus Steam

Steam for Eye Imbalances

Leaf: Calendula, Thyme

Recipe: Sinus Steam

Eye Wash with Eye Cup for Eye Imbalances

Fennel/Comfrey Root Decoction

Calendula Infusion

Lower Respiratory: Lungs

Herbs that are specific to the lungs

Pulmonary: Elecampane, Mullein, Licorice, Hyssop, Coltsfoot, Osha

Anti-microbial: Garlic, Echinacea, Elecampane, Thyme,
Oregon Grape Root

Expectorant: Elder, Plantain

Demulcent: Marshmallow Root, Plantain, Licorice, Slippery Elm,
Irish Moss, Comfrey

Anti-spasmodic: Peppermint, Spearmint

Anticatarrh: Coltsfoot, Hyssop, Goldenrod, Goldenseal, Elder

Antitussive: Wild Cherry Bark

Lungs supply the body with oxygen and dispose of the carbon dioxide which
the body produces as a waste product. This process, known as respiration,

supplies the body with oxygen which it then combines with blood sugar to create the fuel that our cells burn for energy. The lungs are organs of assimilation as well as elimination. Plants do the opposite: they breathe in carbon dioxide and release oxygen.

Proper breathing and the quality of the air that we breathe is essential for our health. In traditional Chinese medicine or TCM the lungs are considered the recipient of chi, or life force. According to the Ayurvedic or Indian tradition, the breath is the vehicle of prana, the universal life force.

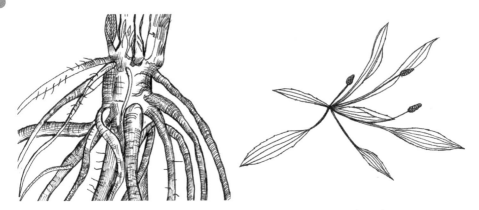

Marshmallow Root (left), Plantain Narrow Leaf (right)

Pulmonary Herbs

Pulmonary herbs work as tonics to the lungs, helping soothe and heal lung imbalances. They might also have other actions that benefit the lungs such as relaxing or stimulating the lungs, helping them get better.

Pulmonaries

Leaf: Mullein, Comfrey*, Coltsfoot*, Tulsi, Plantain

Root: Elecampane, Marshmallow

*Coltsfoot and Comfrey

There is controversy about the herbs Comfrey and Coltsfoot. There herbs have been used for centuries to correct lung imbalances. Check out any herbal books and these are the herbs you will find listed as effective lung tonics.

Recently (as in the last thirty years) they have been vilified because they have been found to contain an alkaloid that is considered to be harmful to the liver. Comfrey and Coltsfoot contain the constituent pyrrolizidine alkaloid or PA's. It was found that consuming pyrrolizidine alkaloids in very large quantities creates a liver imbalance. The case studies are inconclusive but coltsfoot and comfrey received a reputation for being harmful.

Coltsfoot and Comfrey use is limited to specific conditions. They are not herbs that are used as food supplements therefore the amounts would not be harmful as indicated by the studies.

Over the years I have watched many beneficial plants receive bad press. It is important to read the scientific studies about particular maligned plants and increase your knowledge about the process of destroying a plant's reputation to heal. Studies on particular plants are readily available via an internet search.

Because of the controversy, I started substituting marshmallow root for comfrey root and I found that it was a great herb that grows extremely well here. I harvest both the leaves and the root and use them in all sorts of herbal remedies. Marshmallow is a demulcent like comfrey root. I use comfrey root externally in my skin remedies.

I use mullein, elecampane for coughs instead of coltsfoot. I used a combination of herbs for coughs and each imbalance is different so I will use different combination for different people.

Plantain is a popular plant for lung imbalances in Europe. They use the narrow leaf Plantain species. I mention this plant because it has a history of respiratory use.

Plantain has a drawing action and it works in a cough medicine as an expectorant.

Expectorants

Expectorant herbs help the body move the unwanted mucus of the lungs. These plants range from mild to strong. Mild expectorants work gently with the body, helping to expel excess and infected mucus while soothing and healing lung tissue. Strong expectorants do their job by irritating the lungs to stimulate the expectorant process.

Learning to use the right herbs for various conditions is essential, as using strong herbs in a situation can make the condition worse rather than better. This

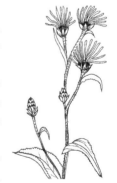

Elecampane

85

was illustrated to me by a friend who, upon contracting a cold and stuffy nose, decided to take a Chinese herbal formula that a friend had given her because her friend had taken it for her cold and it worked great. She took the formula and went to the movies. She started coughing and kept coughing. By the time she called me, the cough had calmed down. As we determined her symptoms and the proper treatment for her cold, we came to the conclusion that she didn't have such a bad cough but that she had taken an herbal formula that was too strong an expectorant: the coughing was induced by the formula. Unfortunately, she had taken another dose of the Chinese medicine before she called me and her strong coughing continued all night long, preventing her from having a restful night sleep (which she needed because she was not well). She had a runny nose but no symptoms that required a strong expectorant.

It is important to know what actions the herbs produce and to match them to your symptoms. An herbal remedy that works for one person doesn't necessarily work for another person.

I have also found that the expectorant action of herbs varies in individuals. Some people are very sensitive to expectorant herbs. Some people take them and the herbs act like tonics. The herbal books are also confusing. Many plants are classified as expectorants when they are really work as antitussives, which means that the herbs quiet or sedate a cough instead of promoting one.

When using and suggesting expectorant herbs, use a small dosage at first and monitor how the individual reacts with the herbs. Increase the dosage if the herbs are working. Many of the herbs labeled as expectorants work as tonics to heal the lungs. These herbs have been employed as remedies from the beginning of time and they work the same in today's world.

My favorite lung herb is elecampane root. It grows wild in the Adirondacks, but I grow it in my garden to ensure a supply. The root has a wonderful smell and taste when it is freshly harvested. The smell and taste get stronger as it ages. I include it in my strong Throat and Chest Decoction remedy. But using it with the addition of my other favorite all-around plant, marshmallow root, makes an all-over effective lung tonic. (Throw a bit of licorice root in for flavor and antimicrobial action, and add a teaspoon of honey and you are good to go.) Those two plants are the ones I think of immediately when dealing with any kind of lung imbalance. As you can see, most herbs share many classifications or actions. Elecampane is an expectorant, demulcent and antimicrobial at once.

Expectorants

Leaf/Flower: Mullein, Horehound, Hyssop, Coltsfoot, Plantain, Elder Blossoms

Root: Elecampane, Licorice, Osha

There are different types of coughs: coughs that are trying to expel mucous in the lungs, coughs caused by sinuses that drain into the lungs (a post nasal dripping that irritates the throat and voice box, and irritating dry coughs caused by environmental issues or allergies. These are just some cough types.

Congested Coughs

Infusions for Congested Coughs

Leaf/Flower: Nettles, Peppermint, Mullein, Catnip, Tulsi, Hyssop, Plantain, Horehound

Recipe: Breathe Easy, Sinus Clearing Remedy

Decoctions for Congested Coughs

Root: Marshmallow Root, Elecampane Root

Recipe: Throat/Chest Decoction, Children's Respiratory Blend

Tinctures for Congested Coughs

Peppermint, Thyme, Yarrow, Echinacea, Goldenseal

Honey Infusion for Congested Coughs

Honey/Garlic Infusion

Syrups for Congested Coughs

Root: Elderberry, Ginger

Recipe: Throat/Chest Decoction

NOTE: Put 1 teaspoon of concentrated syrups into infusions or decoctions for flavoring and effectiveness. I put 1 teaspoon of elderberry syrup into a cup of tulsi tea for a preventative remedy.

External Therapies

Steam for Congested Coughs

Leaf: Thyme, Rosemary

Recipe: Sinus Steam Remedy

Baths/Foot Baths for Congested Coughs

Leaf: Thyme, Yarrow, Catnip

Recipe: Cleansing Bath

Additional

Heating Pads for Congested Coughs

Warm Air Humidifier/Vaporizer

Essential oils of lavender or rosemary for the medicine cup.

Caution: The essential oil of eucalyptus is stimulating to many individuals so I do not recommend using it in a sickroom. Children are particularly affected by eucalyptus.

Dry Coughs

Dry coughs should be treated with herbs that have a demulcent action. Demulcent herbs are soothing to the mucous membranes of the lungs. Strong expectorant herbs are not indicated because the cough is not productive, or helping the lungs expel mucous.

If the cough is interfering with sleep an antitussive herb would help sedate the cough thereby helping the person sleep.

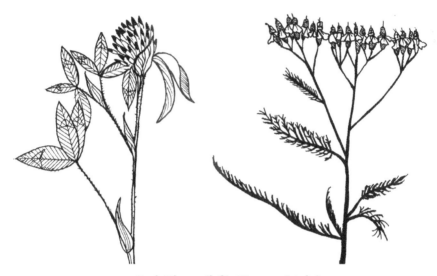

Red Clover (left), Yarrow (right)

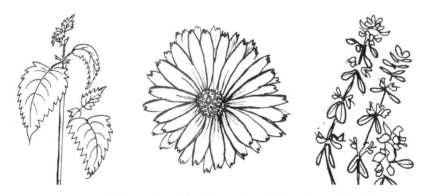

Catnip (left), Calendula flower (middle), Thyme (right)

SECTION 1 | *Get Well*

Infusion for Dry Cough

Leaf: Red Clover Blossoms, Oats, Chamomile, Nettles, Calendula
Recipe: Dry Cough Remedy, Respiratory Clearing Remedy, Sinus Clearing Remedy

Decoction for Dry Cough

Root: Marshmallow Root

Tincture for Dry Cough

Thyme, Echinacea

Syrup for a Dry Cough

Marshmallow, Elderberry, Licorice, Slippery Elm

Honey Infusion for a Dry Cough

Honey/Garlic

Steams for a Dry Cough

Leaf: Thyme
Recipe: Sinus Steam

Baths/Foot Baths for a Dry Cough

Leaf: Yarrow, Catnip

Recipe: Cleansing Bath

Additional

Humidifier

Calming a Cough

A dry or irritating cough can prevent a good night's sleep, especially for children. Wild Cherry Bark sedates the cough reflex which is appropriate to use when the coughing reflex is not productive to the lungs. Demulcent herbs help soothe and protect lung tissues.

Decoction to sedate or quiet a cough

Root: Wild Cherry Bark, Marshmallow

Recipe: Quiet the Cough

Syrup to sedate or quiet a cough

Quiet the Cough

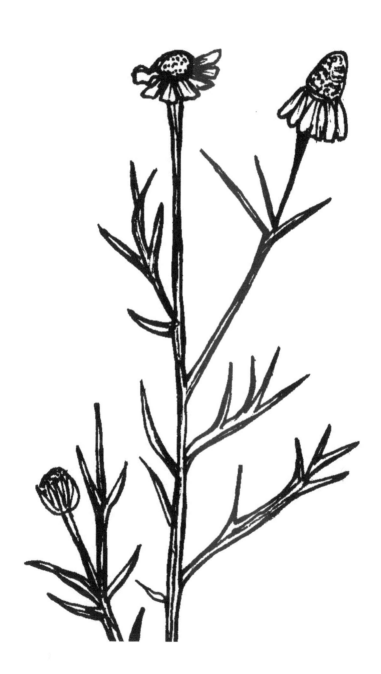

Chapter 11

THE ROLE OF THE DIGESTIVE SYSTEM

The digestive system is a complex system that is the basis for our health. Between the mouth and anus is a complicated set of actions geared to take in food, break food down into minute particles or molecules of nutrients, and absorb such nutrients into the body to create the fuel and energy needed to function. The lower digestive tract breaks down the food we don't use and removes the waste by the peristaltic action of the lower digestive tract muscles.

When we are feeling sick there are many philosophies about what food ought to be consumed. "Feed a cold and stave a fever" is a common adage that makes a lot of sense. When the body is fighting a fever it does not need to work very hard to digest heavy food. Most people with fevers do not feel like eating anyway. Children will not eat (a concern of most mothers). The body needs liquids which are easy to absorb. Tonic herbs are suited for feeding the body the nutrients it needs.

Slippery Elm Root Decoction has been used for centuries as a "gruel" or nutritional tonic when suffering from an illness. It possesses concentrated nutrients and functions as a demulcent to soothe the digestive tract. Peppermint and Chamomile contain strong volatile oils that are antimicrobial to help fight the infection of illness, as well as help the digestive system to function.

Actions of the Herbs for the Digestive System

Tonic herbs help nourish the body by providing nutrients in an absorbable form. When we are sick we do not feel like eating but an herbal infusion or decoction can provide some necessary nutrients to retrieve our much-needed energy.

Leaf: Oats, Tulsi

Root: Marshmallow, Licorice

Bark: Slippery Elm

Demulcent herbs soothe and protect the mucous membranes, particularly the walls of the digestive tract. They lubricate the gastrointestinal tract while providing added nutrients.

Leaf: Oats

Root: Marshmallow Root, Licorice

Bark: Slippery Elm

Bitters are herbs that have a bitter taste and promote better digestion. Although the role of bitters is really a subject for another book, herbal remedies that contain special bitter digestive herbs can be found in the traditional medicine of Europe, India and China.

Bitter herbs help tonify and strengthen the digestion and nervous system. They activate the gastric secretion of hydrochloric acid and other digestive enzymes. They specifically help the liver in its role as detoxifier. The bitter taste in the mouth activates the whole response of the digestive system, helping it do its job. Many of the traditional "sick" herbs are very bitter which I am sure helps the liver process the toxins that come with fighting an illness.

One of the most popular bitter formulas is "Swedish Bitters". It is an ancient herbal formula that was rediscovered by an Austrian herbalist named Maria Treben. She tells the story of bitters and of people's experiences using them in her book, *Health through God's Pharmacy*. An acquaintance of mine who owned a health food store over twenty years ago told me that for several years after closing her store she still ordered "Swedish Bitters" for her elderly customers because they worked so well. Bitters are helpful to restart the digestive processes after an illness. They are taken thirty minutes before mealtimes to stimulate the appetite and get all the juices flowing.

Flower: Chamomile

Leaf: Chicory

Root: Dandelion, Burdock, Gentian, Artichoke, Angelica

Peel: Orange peel

Carminatives are plants that contain aromatic volatile oils that stimulate the gastrointestinal tract to do its job. Small plates of anise, cardamom and other types of seeds are served as an after-dinner snack at my local Indian restaurant. Crunching these carminative seeds after a meal helps you to digest.

Leaf/Flower: Peppermint, Ginger, Chamomile, Spearmint

Bark: Cinnamon

Seed: Fennel, Dill, Anise, Cardamom

Anti-Spasmodics relax the muscles to prevent cramping. They are useful for alleviating stomach and intestinal cramping. Peppermint is a specific for intestinal cramps.

Leaf/Flower: Chamomile, Peppermint, Motherwort, Skullcap

Root: Valerian Root

Bark: Cramp Bark

Peppermint, Fennel Seed, Ginger, Chamomile

Four main herbs work well for imbalances of the digestive system. These plants seem to be the workhorses for what ails people most. Just like there are different sorts of people, there are peppermint people and there are fennel people: these plants appeal to different people and when they find their digestive plant they are happy campers. I have found that these plants all appeal to different people.

Indigestion

Indigestion can be caused by any number of things. I am focusing on basic digestive issues that one is likely to encounter when sick.

Infusions for Indigestion

Leaf: Peppermint, Spearmint, Chamomile
Seed: Fennel
Recipe: Digest & Rest

Decoctions for Indigestion

Root: Ginger, Marshmallow, Licorice
Bark: Slippery Elm Bark
Seed: Fennel
Recipe: Smooth Digestion, G I Tonic

Syrups for Indigestion

Ginger Root

Tinctures for Indigestion

Peppermint, Chamomile

Cramping

Infusions for Cramping

Leaf: Peppermint, Spearmint
Seed: Fennel

Decoctions for Cramping

Root: Ginger

Bark: Cinnamon, Cramp bark

Syrups for Cramping

Ginger

Tinctures for Cramping

Peppermint, Chamomile, Cramp Bark

Nausea

Post nasal drip causes stomach problems.

Infusion for Nausea

Leaf: Peppermint, Chamomile, Red Raspberry Leaf, Spearmint

Seed: Fennel

Recipe: Digest & Rest

Decoction for Nausea

Root: Ginger, Marshmallow Root

Recipe: Smooth Digestion, GI Tonic

Syrups for Nausea

Ginger

Tincture for Nausea

Peppermint, Chamomile

Diarrhea

Diarrhea is a common symptom of the cold and flu. The problem usually corrects itself in several days. With diarrhea, you want to be sure that you get enough fluids into the system, particularly for children. Since the body is ridding itself of infection, it is not productive to stop this action. You can use several herbs to restore the digestive tract, like demulcent herbs which soothe inflamed tissues and bring the system back to normal. Antibiotics might cause diarrhea, so it is wise to take a probiotic supplement or eat yogurt while taking antibiotics.

Infusion for Diarrhea

Leaf: Red Raspberry Leaf, Chamomile, Meadowsweet

Decoctions for Diarrhea

Root: Marshmallow

Bark: Slippery Elm, Cinnamon

Tincture for Diarrhea

Goldenseal

Grapefruit Seed Extract

Vomiting

Vomiting, like diarrhea, is a symptom associated with colds and the flu. It cleans out the stomach in a hurry which can be a good thing. Again, the concern is that vomiting can lead to dehydration, especially in children. Drinking any liquid (especially large quantities) will trigger the vomiting reflex so take liquid in very small amounts after each episode of vomiting. Herbs that are helpful for nausea and diarrhea are appropriate for calming the stomach.

The "brat diet" helps restore the digestive tract back to normal. The letters stand for Bananas, Rice, Applesauce, and Toast. While faced with what to eat after a bout with the intestinal flu or cold these foods are a good start. Of course, soup broths are in order as well.

Electrolytes Replacement Drink

1 cup warm or room temperature water

1 pinch baking soda

1 pinch salt

1 tablespoon honey, maple syrup or sugar

Substitute herbal infusion for water: try Spearmint,
Chamomile or Fennel Seed Infusions.

This combination of ingredients replaces the balance of minerals in the body which might be disturbed by episodes of vomiting or diarrhea. Putting salt, sugars, and bicarbonate soda into herbal teas is a good way to help the body get better.

Chapter 12

ROLE OF THE NERVOUS SYSTEM

The nervous system is our gateway to the outside world. It helps us perceive and deal with what we encounter. We use our five senses of taste, sight, hearing, touch and smell to engage the world and we respond through the fabric of our nervous system. It is an electric system, moving energy through the billions of cells embedded into every fiber of our being. But bodies are so much more than electrical biochemical machines. Plants that work in conjunction with our nervous systems are so valuable to helping us negotiate the world.

Herbs that impact the nervous system are the most sought-after plants in the world. This is such a maligned group of plants because of the way people have used or abused these plants throughout history. A perfect example is the recent history of the marijuana plant. This plant was outlawed in the 1930s. At the time, the government reinstated the legality of alcohol but created a ban on the cannabis plant. In the United States today, we are becoming aware of the incredible healing properties of this plant but it is still illegal on the federal level, which considers cannabis to be a "substance 1" drug. Cannabis is not a drug but a plant. This plant has been altered from its original form by cultivating the plants with the highest concentrations of THC. THC constituent has a much-desired psychoactive effect on the nervous system. Along with the poppy plant and the cocoa plant of South America, plants that alter consciousness and the state of the nervous system have been used throughout history.

There are so many other plants that should have their place in our world of herbal apothecary besides the cannabis plant. The plant world is brimming with plants that help our nervous systems stay healthy and balanced. Because of the total misuse of this category of plants, people are hesitant to use other nervous system herbs—a terrible shame given that when used properly they are a gift to mankind.

Plant irony

When I first started learning about medicinal plants forty years ago, the only "herb" people knew about was marijuana. Now it seems I am back to square one. But this time, the plant in question is becoming known for its incredible medicinal qualities rather than its sedative or psychoactive qualities. So I believe that cannabis or marijuana will be this country's gateway "plant" to the popular use of botanical medicine, rather than a gateway "drug" to other drugs that destroy rather than heal a person.

Nervine Herbal Actions

These plants can help when faced with an acute illness to:

- *Alleviate stress:* Chamomile - nervine
- *Calm and relax the body*: Passionflower - relaxant
- *Cope with pain:* Valerian Root - analgesic
- *Boost much-needed energy during recovery*: Ginger - stimulant
- *Keep the body well*: Astragalus - adaptagen

Find the Plant that Works for You

The plants that impact our nervous system are véry individualized. People react differently to these plants so it is wise to be cautious with the dosage when trying out different plants. Finding a plant that helps one relax or sleep is a gift and I recommend getting to know these plants before you get sick.

My Favorite Nervines

Valerian root is my go-to plant of choice for sleeping. I have always said that it got me through my kids' teenage years. But when I started to work with clients I found that it was too strong for many people. Some people found it to be too sedating, so much so that they were still groggy in the morning (the opposite of my experience: when I use it, I sleep better and I feel rested in the morning). It also has a quirk in that a small percentage of the population will find it to be stimulating rather than sedating. Not a plant you want to recommend to a person who is having trouble sleeping.

I have since found that Passionflower is an all-around wonderful nervine plant for the majority of people. It is relaxing without being too strong. Chamomile falls in my category of being "gentle but strong", too. It is extremely effective for relaxing the body with the added benefit of helping the digestive system. It is a good herb for some children. Again, it is important to try out different plants.

The Versatile Peppermint Plant

One the most interesting and versatile plants I have encountered is peppermint. It contains both a stimulating and relaxing action at the same time. In the herbal world, this is called a "normalizer". The other plant that works this way is tobacco. It relaxes the body while keeping people alert. No wonder is it such a sought after plant. Peppermint serves so many purposes and is a good plant to get to know. It is extremely helpful when treating acute illnesses: it helps the respiratory system soothe the lungs, it helps the digestive system relax and digest, and it can be a good plant to put into an herbal recipe to liven it up both with flavor and an uplifting quality.

Some people find peppermint to be too strong but love spearmint, another member of the mint family. Spearmint has similar but gentler actions. Both plants are prolific here in the Northeast and should be added to your list of plants to grow and know.

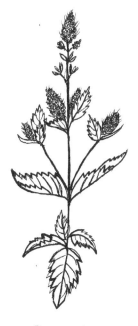

Peppermint

Actions of Cold and Flu Herbs for the Nervous System

"Nervine" is a term that describes herbs that strengthen and calm the nervous system of the body. They are high in specific nutrients that feed the nervous system. Some herbs work gently to restore and balance our body similar to a tonic action. Other plants have a much stronger sedating action which enables us to relax and get the sleep that we need while ill. Sleep is so important in the healing process. We have been taught to push through an illness instead of taking the time to care for ourselves. Nervines help to relax us, which in integral to getting better.

I tend to use the term "nervine" to describe any plant that has an effect on the nervous system. Stimulating herbs have their place in helping the body heal as well. First, we start with the actions of the calming herbs.

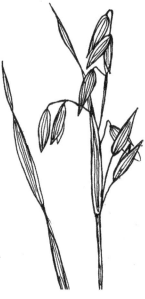

Oat Plant

Sedative herbs

Sedative herbs refers to plants that calm and relax the nervous system. They range in action from calming to strong sedation. Different nervous systems respond differently to nervine plants; I highly recommend finding the nervine plants that work for you. These plants are a gift in a stressful world but can be particularly useful when trying to calm the body in order to heal from an illness.

Gentle Sedatives

Leaf/Flower: Chamomile, Catnip, Lemon Balm, Wood Betony, Lavender, Oats, Roses

Stronger Sedatives

Leaf/Flower: Passionflower, Skullcap, California Poppy

Root: Valerian

Stimulant herbs

Stimulant herbs fall on the other end of the nervine plant spectrum. These plants increase the body's metabolism. They give the body energy. They are appropriate for use during the recovery phase of an illness. Coffee is a perfect example of an herb that stimulates the whole body. Coffee was originally used as medicine to help people recover from illnesses because it gave them a boost of energy which they needed after being sick.

Cayenne, ginger and peppermint also work as stimulants. For instance, I include cayenne in my cold cap/yellow pill powder. It gives a needed boost of energy to the formula so that the pills work faster in the body. The cayenne helps move the herbs through the body at a faster pace. It unsticks the metabolism. I have tried the pills without the

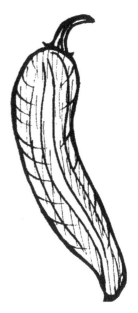

Cayenne

cayenne in them and I didn't think that they worked as well. Sometimes the body gets stuck in a pattern and just needs a little boost to start improving. Stimulant herbs help move the cold or flu through its paces so that one gets better faster.

Stimulant herbs:

Leaf/Flower: Peppermint, Yerba Matte, Coffee, Black Tea, Green Tea

Root: Ginger, Siberian ginseng (Eleutherococcus), American ginseng, Panax ginseng

Fruit: Cayenne

The key thing to remember is that true energy is derived from nutritional food and not by using stimulating herbs. Soups and easy-to-digest meals are necessary for regaining the energy in the body after an illness.

Analgesic herbs

Analgesic herbs are plants that help relieve pain. Sometimes we cannot rest because we are feeling terrible from the flu. It is essential that we sleep to recover and sometimes we can't because we are in pain.

"Take two aspirin and call me in the morning" is an adage that translates to something like this: You are going to get better anyway, it's just the flu: take a pain reliever so that you can sleep and you'll feel better in the morning.

It is important to address the aches and pains of the flu and colds, though, and for this purpose this category of herbs is very helpful.

Analgesic herbs

Leaf/Flower: Passionflower, Chamomile, Skullcap, Meadowsweet, Peppermint, Catnip, St. John's Wort

Root: Valerian

Bark: Willow

Anti-inflammatory herbs

Anti-inflammatory herbs soothe inflammations of the body. Although inflammations occur in many instances, inflamed tissues can be a symptom of colds and flu (such as a swollen, sore throat). Reducing inflammation reduces pain.

Anti-inflammatory herbs:

Leaf/Flower: Calendula, Chamomile, Meadowsweet, Yarrow, St. John's Wort

Bark: Willow

Root: Turmeric, Ginger, Licorice

Headaches

Headaches are caused by a variety of imbalances. This book is concerned with headaches that are caused by acute illnesses such as colds and the flu. Sinus headaches are a very common and very painful condition of congested sinuses. A headache might precede a cold or the flu. I would suggest sleeping as a first resort and then using herbs to relax and de-stress the body. Wood Betony is a relaxant of the first order and is considered a specific for headaches. It is not a sedative and I like to combine it with nutritional herbs. External therapies are so effective for relaxing the body, too: a steam for the sinuses is very useful for alleviating the pain of a sinus headache or any other headache. It is my first treatment of choice for along with the appropriate teas.

Infusions for Headaches

Leaf/Flower: Wood Betony, Tulsi, Chamomile, Peppermint, Meadowsweet

Recipe: Healthy Head

Decoctions for Sinus Headaches

Roots: Turmeric, Ginger

Recipe: Throat Health

Powder/Capsules for Sinus Headaches

Cold Caps/Yellow Pills

External Therapy for Headaches

Steam Inhalation: Sinus Steam

Poultice for Headaches

Ginger

Essential Oil

Lavender essential oil diluted with carrier oil rubbed on forehead

Bath/Foot Bath for Headaches

Relax Bath

Pain

Pain all over the body—particularly in the joints—is a common symptom of the flu. Inflammation causes pain. A throat which is swollen and in-flamed can be extremely painful. It is important to address the underlying cause with appropriate herbs, then use herbs to help alleviate the pain. Willow bark has been used for centuries for pain. Aspirin was developed from the bark of the willow tree.

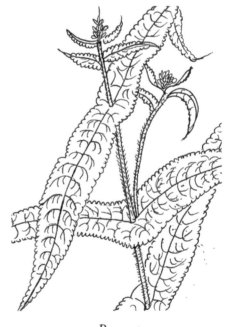

Boneset

Infusion for Pain

Infusion: Boneset- specific plant for body aches of the flu. Chamomile, Valerian, Skullcap, Passionflower, Peppermint, Catnip, Meadowsweet, St. John's Wort

Recipe: Traditional Gypsy Flu Remedy

Decoction for Pain

Bark: Willow bark

Root: Kava

Tincture for Pain

Valerian, Skullcap, Chamomile, Willow Bark, Passionflower, Meadowsweet, St. John's Wort, Cayenne, Kava

Powder/Capsules for Pain

Valerian, Willow Bark, Passionflower, Meadowsweet, Kava, Turmeric

External Therapies for Pain

Essential Oil

Lavender- dilute with carrier oil before using.

Herbal Oils and Ointment for Pain

St. John's Wort oil for muscle pain

Arnica oil for muscle pain

Cayenne ointment

Baths/Foot Baths for Pain

Leaf: Chamomile, Oats

Recipe: Relax Bath

Additional

Heating pads

Cold Sores

Cold sores are caused by the herpes virus 1 which affects the nerve endings of the cells. Please see the **Respiratory** section for further information about dealing with the pain of cold sores.

Anxiety/Calming/Sleeping

Anxiety is a common byproduct of becoming ill. Pain creates anxiety. When we can't sleep and need to sleep while we are sick, nervine herbs can help calm the anxious feeling about giving up the "to do" list that so often keeps many (especially women) awake. The body needs to take a break. The herbs that help anxiousness

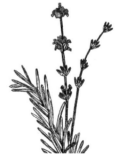

Lavender

also help the body relax. Consider using these plants along with healing plants when facing an illness. Some of the strong cold and flu plants such as catnip also contain a calming action. The herb Kava is considered to be a specific for anxiety. These herbs work well by themselves or combined with other nervine herbs. The gentle sedative herbs are sometimes all that is necessary to ensure a good night's sleep and take the edge off an anxious condition.

Infusion for Anxiety/Calming/Sleeping

Gentle sedatives:

Leaf/Flower: Chamomile, Catnip, Lemon Balm, Wood Betony, Lavender, Oats, Roses

---

Stronger sedatives:

Leaf/Flower: Passionflower, Skullcap, California Poppy

Root: Valerian

Powder/Capsules for Anxiety/Calming/Sleeping

Gentle sedatives:

Leaf/Flower: Chamomile, Catnip, Lemon Balm, Wood Betony, Oats

---

Stronger sedatives:

Leaf: Passionflower, Skullcap, California Poppy

Root: Kava, Valerian

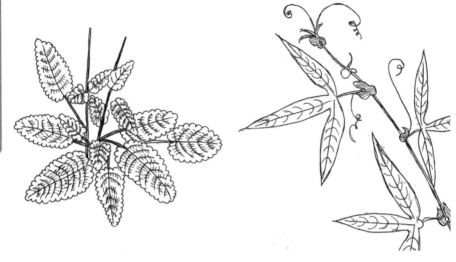

Wood Betony (left), Passionflower (right)

Tinctures for Anxiety/Calming/Sleeping

Gentle sedatives:

Leaf/Flower: Chamomile, Catnip, Lemon Balm, Wood Betony, Oats

---

Stronger sedatives:

Leaf: Passionflower, Skullcap, Valerian Root, California Poppy

Root: Kava

External Therapies

Bath/Foot Bath

Leaf: Chamomile, Oats

Recipe: Relax Bath

Additional

Heating pads

The Role of Nervine Herbs in Recovery

The category of herbs that helps people regain their energy after an illness contains herbs that stimulate the nervous system rather than sedate it. Just as a lack of energy is probably the first sign of the onset of an illness, it is the last symptom to go as we start to get well.

Coffee was originally used as an herbal stimulant. It helped people regain their energy after an illness. As a matter of fact, I know of many, many people who use coffee's stimulating qualities every day to boost their energy. Stimulant herbs are best used once you are in the recovery phase.

Remember (as I have stated over and over): the true source of energy is good nutrition. The tonic herbs that are loaded with nutrients are the go-to herbs for recovery. Plants that help remove unwanted toxins from the body are also helpful in the recovery phase.

- Stimulant herbs give the body energy
- Stimulant herbs boost the effectiveness of an herbal recipe
- Tonic herbs supply much-needed nutrition to give the body energy

Nutritional Infusions for Recovery

Leaf/Flower: Nettles, Oats, Green Tea,
Peppermint, Tulsi

Recipe: Nutritional Everyday Blend,
Favorite Preventative Blend, Three Lemon Tea,
Cheri's Recipe, Uplift

Decoctions for Recovery

Root: Burdock Root, Licorice, Ginger Root

Bark: Siberian Ginseng

Recipe: Energy Root Blend,

Syrups for Recovery

Ginger, Elderberry, Energy Root Blend

Powders/Capsules for Recovery

Root: Turmeric, Ginger

Green Nutritional Powder

Energy Powder

Liver Tonic

Tinctures for Recovery

Burdock Root, Siberian Ginseng

Food for Recovery

Bone Broth Soups, Greens, Oatmeal

External Therapies

Bath

Relax Bath, Cleansing Bath

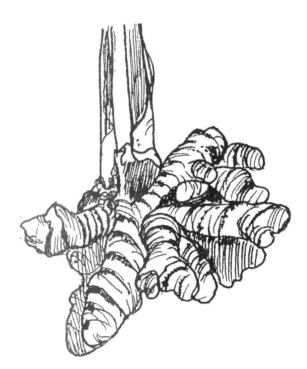

Tumeric Root

Ginseng Root

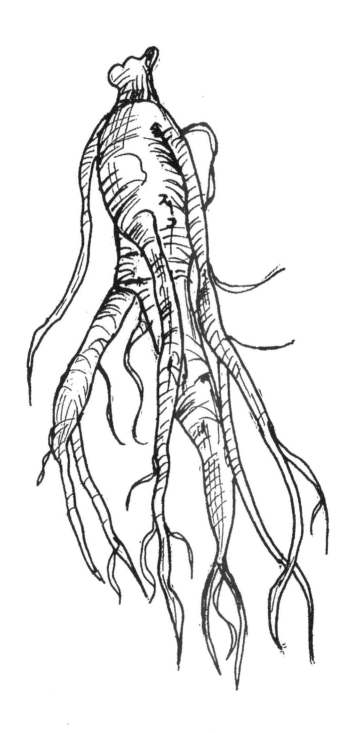

Chapter 13

THE ROLE OF THE IMMUNE SYSTEM

Our immune system's job is to ward off organisms that are harmful to the intricate workings of the body. Current thinking considers the skin, lymphatic system, spleen, thymus, bone marrow, tonsils/adenoids and the appendix to be the immune system organs that play a major role in keeping us healthy and whole. Until a few years ago, the tonsils, adenoids and appendix were considered to be useless organs and were routinely removed. Today we understand that they play a role in the immunity of the body. The emergence of AIDS and other autoimmune diseases has changed the way that scientists look at the immune system. Autoimmune diseases occur when the body regards its own tissues as foreign and mounts an immunity attack against them.

For the purpose of this book we will discuss the immune system's quick or acute response to a cold or viral illness such as the flu. I think of the immune system as comprised of two different systems: the acute system and the long-term system. They have two different jobs. The acute immune system kicks in when the body faces an immediate viral, bacterial, or fungal threat. The long-term immune system keeps us healthy in the long-term and helps protect us from getting sick in the first place. The herbs that help us maintain a good long-term immune system or robust health are revered throughout history. The plant kingdom is overflowing with herbs that help us through acute illnesses as well as herbs that help maintain our health long-term.

Homeostasis

Our bodies are physically geared towards being healthy. The term homeostasis describes the body's natural inclination to achieve a healthy and whole state of being. When we have a cold or the flu, we realize that we need to give our bodies some time to recover. The body systems all work together as a whole to become well again. Herbal plants help move the body into a wholeness state in a balanced way. Rather than suppressing the symptoms of an illness, herbal plants boost the actions of body systems to do their job. Adaptagen herbs are very helpful in helping the body regain its health.

Adaptagen Herbs

This relatively new category of plants helps the body cope with stress. The terminology may be new but the use of these plants is ancient. They work as tonics to all body systems, especially the immune system. These plants are taken not during an acute illness but rather before or after an illness to keep the body stay strong so that you are not susceptible to every illness that seems to appear out of nowhere during the winter season. Getting better and staying better is a big concern of many people as their health tends to be vulnerable after they have recovered from an illness. These plants are used long term to maintain the health and wellbeing of the body. They are very helpful during the winter season.

The terms "adaptagenic medicine" and "adaptagen plants" were first coined by a Russian scientist and pharmacologist, N. V. Laxarev. He sought to describe plants that helped the entire body cope with stress, bringing the body back to homeostasis without any physical side effects. Later, a Swedish scientist, Dr. Hans Selve, explored the major role that stress plays in our lives and our physical bodies. He termed a disorder called "General Adaptive Syndrome" during his research. He explained that the most important factor in bodily health was the body's ability to manage stressful situations. How we react to stressful situations, he explained, is more important to our health than the nature of the stressors that we encounter in life. How we cope with stress is completely individual.

Although they are not recognized by the mainstream medical system, adaptagens have been revered throughout history. For example, the Asian herb, Panax ginseng, and the American herb, Panax quinquefolius, are such sought-after plants that they demand huge prices in the international herb trade markets. The ginseng plants with which people are most familiar have adaptive-type actions. Lesser-known is the Eleutherococcus bush, which was given the common name "Siberian ginseng" to link its adaptagen qualities to the more famous ginseng plant.

Eleuthero

The Eleuthero plant has an interesting history. Siberian ginseng (Eleutheroccus senticosus) is not a true ginseng but a woody shrub from eastern Siberia that shares the same plant family, Aralia. It is related to a North American species called American spikenard (Aralia racemosa), Hercule's Club (Aralia spinosa) and a very common plant that grows prolifically in the woods around here: Wild sarsaparilla (Aralia nudicaulis). A Russian scientist, I. Brekman, studied plants from the Aralia family to see if other species shared some of the healing qualities of the American and Asian ginsengs. He found that the Eleuthero plant did indeed have similar qualities. He named it Siberian ginseng to connect its adaptagen attributes in people's minds even though it was not in the same genus as the other ginsengs. It is a highly studied and researched plant that is very helpful during the recovery phase of an illness and as a stimulating tonic to help the body cope with stress. It can be taken much longer than other ginseng plants: its actions are different from the stronger ginseng plants in protecting the body from stressors long term. It was used by the 1984 Moscow Olympics athletes. The Russians were very interested in the adaptagen plants role in improving athletic performances. There is much research about the Russian's use of adaptagens in their sports programs.

The decoction, tincture and ground powder of Siberian ginseng help you recover from an illness. These preparations also help people cope with the day-to-day stresses that come their way.

I combine Siberian ginseng, burdock and marshmallow roots to create an uplifting decoction to be taken as one is recovering from an illness and needs an extra boost of energy.

Ginseng

There are two types of ginseng available. The Asian ginseng, Panax ginseng, is the most popular ginseng plant. In the East, ginseng is the panacea for all types of health conditions; many ginseng preparations exist, including ginseng chewing gum. In the United States, an American species, Panax quin-quefolius, grows or used to grow in the Adirondacks and Catskill mountains. However, nowadays it is rarely found in the wild: a mainstay of American export to Asia since settlers arrived in the 1700s, the plant has become a victim of over-harvesting.

If you do find a wild ginseng plant, please do not dig it up just because you can. The majority of people who feel the need to harvest wild ginseng only do so because they know it is rare and valuable: often, they have no idea how to use it or to whom they should sell it. I have received too many phone calls from people who have harvested the plant to make a quick buck. Many know that it is a "valuable" plant worth lots of money—but that's as deep as their understanding goes. When you dig up a plant for its roots you kill the plant: those who harvest ginseng just for its projected value will waste its potential benefits.

There are many cultivated ginsengs on the market. For further research into growing this plant and other woodland plants, check out *Growing and Marketing Ginseng, Goldenseal and Other Woodland Medicinals* by Jeanine Davis and W. Scott Persons

American Ginseng

American ginseng is helpful when used in the recovery phase of an illness, as well as when taken as a general tonic. It gives one energy, bringing the body back into balance. It is considered to be less strong than the Panax species, but is still well-suited for recovery and energy-boosting. In fact, most people I know prefer it to the stronger Asian ginseng species.

Rhodiola rosa

The species *Rhodiola rosa* grows in the higher altitudes of Russia, Asia, and Scandinavia. In those parts of the world, it was used for centuries in traditional medicines. Other Rhodiola species originate in other parts of the world, including North America. The rosa species is medicinal in na-ture, so be sure to accurately identify the species before using this plant. It has been extensively studied as an adaptagen and there is much litera-ture available about its ability to improve athletic performance, reduce fatigue, combat high-altitude sickness, alleviate depression, and mitigate other health problems. I combine rhodiola powder with turmeric powder to make a protective, energy-boosting capsule that helps my body deal with cold winters.

Astragalus

Astragalus comes from the Traditional Chinese Medicine (TCM) tradition. The Chinese use it in combination with other herbs to help the body stay healthy. The root is prepared by way of a special process; when you purchase it, it looks like a tongue depressor. I use the root in my soups to enhance the power of the healing qualities of the food.

Fungi

We can thank mycologist Paul Stamets from Washington State for his extensive and comprehensive research about the world of fungi. Through his business Fungi Perfecti (www. fungi.com), Stamets has made all types of mushrooms available for purchase, including mushroom products like grow-your-own mushroom kits. Mushrooms play a huge role in the health of our planet as well as our bodies. Take the time to explore different types of mushrooms for your health and wellbeing.

The Use of Adaptagen Herbs in Recovery

Use adaptagen herbs after you have been ill, but not during the illness itself. It is appropriate to use them as you recover, but no sooner insofar as they work as tonics that support the long-term immune system. They are not appropriate for helping the short-term immune system.

- *Root:* Siberian Ginseng (Eleutherococcus), American Ginseng, Rhodiola, Astragalus, Ashwagandha

- *Mushroom:* Reishi, Fungi Kingdom

- *Recipe:* Energy Root Blend, Energy Powder

The Use of Adaptagen Herbs in Staying Healthy

- ☙ *Root:* Siberian Ginseng, American Ginseng, Astragalus, Rhodiola, Ashwagandha

- ☙ *Berry:* Schizandra

- ☙ *Mushroom:* Reishi, Chaga

- ☙ *Recipe:* Energy Root Blend, Energy Powder

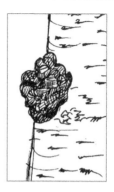

Chaga

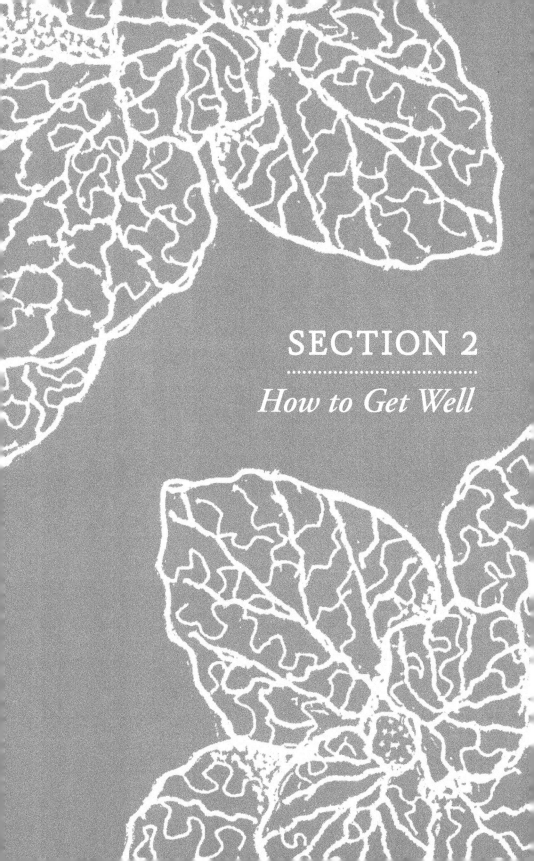

SECTION 2

How to Get Well

Chapter 14
SYMPTOMS

The symptoms are listed alongside the specific herbs and herbal preparations that are used for the symptoms you are experiencing. Do not become overwhelmed by the many choices. I give a variety of options because the plants work that way and you might have different herbs on hand (especially if you have an herbal garden). Determine what works best for you and then turn to the **Preparation** chapter for directions on how to make the recipes. I have underlined the plants that have a history of being specific for particular problems. You will usually need just one or two preparations. By all means, do not forget to use herbs for external applications, too.

Allergies

See Chapter 6: Cold or Flu or Allergy, page 33.

Treat according to symptoms.

Anxiety

See Chapter 12: The Role of the Nervous System, page 101.

Simple Infusions: Chamomile, Lemon Balm, Wood Betony, Oats, Passionflower

Infusion Recipes: Relaxation Blend, Healthy Head, Digest & Rest, Uplift

Simple Decoctions: Kava

Tinctures: Kava, Passionflower, Valerian

Herbal Steam: Chamomile, Oats, Lavender, Roses, Relax Bath

Herbal Bath: Chamomile, Oats, Relax Bath

Heating Pad

Calming/Relaxation

See Chapter 12: The Role of the Nervous System, page 101.

Simple Infusions: Lemon Balm, Wood Betony, Oats, Catnip, Chamomile, Valerian, Passionflower

Infusion Recipe: Relaxation Blend, Digest & Rest

Simple Decoctions: Kava

Herbal Powders/Capsules: Passionflower, Valerian

Tinctures: Kava, Wood Betony, Passionflower, Chamomile

Herbal Bath: Relax Bath

Hot Pad

Cold Sores/Fever Blisters

See Chapter 10: The Role of the Respiratory System, page 63.

Simple Infusion: Lemon Balm, Calendula

Infusion Recipes: Cold/Sore Infusion

Decoction Recipes: Cold sore Root Blend

Tinctures: Licorice, St. John's Wort, Lemon Balm applied topically

Herbal Oil: St. John's Wort, Lemon Balm applied topically

Poultice: Onion

Coughs

See Chapter 10: The Role of the Respiratory System, page 63.

CHILDREN'S COUGH

Simple Infusions: Catnip, Peppermint, Mullein

Infusion Recipes: Breathe Easy

Honey Infusion: Honey/Garlic

Simple Decoctions: Marshmallow root, Elecampane, Licorice

Decoction Recipes: Children's Respiratory Decoction

Syrups: Elderberry

Poultice: Onion

CONGESTED COUGHS

Simple Infusions: Catnip, Peppermint, Mullein, Hyssop, Horehound, Plantain, Nettles, Tulsi

Infusion Recipes: Breathe Easy, Sinus Clearing Remedy, Congested Cough Infusion

Honey Infusion: Honey/Garlic

Simple Decoctions: Marshmallow root, Elecampane

Decoction Recipes: Throat/Chest Decoction, Children's Respiratory Blend

Syrups: Elderberry, Ginger, Throat/Chest

Vinegar: Honey/Apple Cider, Winter Root

Powders/Capsules: Cold caps, Yellow pills

Tinctures: Peppermint, Yarrow, Thyme, Goldenseal, Echinacea

Steam: Thyme, Rosemary, Sinus Steam

Bath: Catnip, Yarrow, Cleansing Bath

Heating Pad

Humidifier

DRY COUGHS

Simple Infusions: Nettles, Oats, Calendula, Chamomile

Infusion Recipes: Dry Cough Remedy

Honey Infusion: Honey/Garlic

Simple Decoctions: Marshmallow root

Decoction Recipes: Children's Respiratory Blend

Syrups: Marshmallow root, Licorice, Elderberry, Ginger,

Powder/Capsules: Slippery Elm, Cold caps, Yellow pills,

Tinctures: Echinacea, Thyme

Steam: Thyme, Sinus Steam

Bath: Catnip, Yarrow, Cleansing Bath

Heating Pad

Humidifier

CALMING AN IRRITATING COUGH

Simple Decoctions: Wild Cherry Bark

Decoction Recipes: Quiet the Cough

Heating Pad

Poultice: Onion

Humidifier

Cramping

See Chapter 11: The Role of the Digestive System, page 93.

Simple Infusions: Peppermint, Chamomile, Spearmint

Infusion Recipes: Digest & Rest

Simple Decoctions: Marshmallow root, Ginger, Fennel seed

Decoction Recipes: Smooth Digestion, GI Tonic

Syrups: Ginger

Tinctures: Peppermint, Chamomile

Bath: Catnip, Chamomile, Ginger, Cleansing Bath

Heating Pad

Diarrhea

See Chapter 11: The Role of the Digestive System, page 93.

Food: Oatmeal, BRAT diet: Bananas, Rice, Applesauce and Toast

Simple Infusions: Red Raspberry Leaf, Meadowsweet

Simple Decoctions: Slippery Elm Bark, Marshmallow root

Powders: Slippery Elm Bark, Cinnamon

Grapefruit Seed Extract

Earache/Infections

See Chapter 10: The Role of the Respiratory System, page 63.

Simple Infusions: Peppermint, Catnip, Elderberry, Mullein

Infusion Recipes: Breathe Easy, Traditional Gypsy Flu Remedy

Honey Infusion: Honey/Garlic

Simple Decoctions: Marshmallow root, Licorice

Decoction Recipes: Children's Respiratory Blend

Syrups: Elderberry, Ginger, Children's Respiratory Blend

Tinctures: Echinacea, Goldenseal, Thyme, Yarrow

Steam: Thyme, Sinus Steam

Bath: Catnip, Yarrow, Cleansing Bath

Herbal Ear Oil: Garlic or Mullein Flower , Olive oil

Heating Pad

Humidifier

Energy

See Chapter 12: The Role of the Nervous System, page 101.

Simple Infusions: Nettles, Oats, Green Tea, Peppermint, Tulsi

Infusion Recipes: Nutritional Everyday Blend, Favorite Preventative Blend, Children's Preventative Drink

Decoction Recipes: Energy Root Blend

Syrups: Ginger, Energy Root Blend

Herbal Powders/Capsules: Energy Powder, Liver Tonic Powder

Tinctures: Siberian Ginseng

Eye Infections

. . . .

See Chapter 10: The Role of the Respiratory System, page 63.

Simple Infusions: Catnip, Calendula

Infusion Recipes: Eye Imbalance, Congested Cough

Honey Infusion: Honey/Garlic

Simple Decoctions: Elderberry, Marshmallow root, Licorice

Decoction Recipes: Children's Respiratory Blend,

Syrups: Elderberry, Ginger

Vinegar: Honey/Apple Cider, Winter Root Cider

Powders/Capsules: Cold caps, Yellow Pills

Tinctures: Goldenseal, Echinacea

Herbal Eye Wash: Calendula, Fennel seed/Comfrey Root

Humidifier

Fever

. . . .

See Chapter 6: Cold or Flu or Allergy, page 33.
See Chapter 9: Demulcents, page 53.

See herbs for Flu

Fever - Children

. . . .

Simple Infusions: Catnip, Chamomile

Syrups: Elderberry

Tinctures: Echinacea, Echinacea Glycerin

Herbal Steam: Sinus Steam

Herbal Bath: Catnip, Cleansing Bath

Humidifier

Flu Adults

....

See Chapter 6: Cold or Flu or Allergy, page 33.
See Chapter 9: Demulcents, page 53.

Food: Bone Broth, Soup

Simple Infusions: Boneset, Yarrow, Catnip, Elder Flower, Thyme, Chamomile, Peppermint

Infusion Recipes: Traditional Gypsy Flu Remedy

Honey Infusion: Honey/Garlic

Simple Decoctions: Marshmallow root, Licorice

Decoction Recipes: Smooth Digestion

Syrups: Ginger, Elderberry

Herbal Powders/Capsules: Cold caps/Yellow pills

Tinctures: Yarrow, Thyme, Catnip

Steam: Thyme, Sinus Steam

Bath: Yarrow, Catnip, Cleansing Bath

Heating Pads

Humidifier

Headache

....

See Chapter 12: The Role of the Nervous System, page 101.

Simple Infusions: Wood Betony, Chamomile, Peppermint, Tulsi, Meadowsweet

Infusion Recipes: Healthy Head, Sinus Cleaning Remedy, Digest & Rest

Simple Decoction: Turmeric, Ginger

Herbal Powders/Capsules: Turmeric

Tinctures: Wood Betony, Meadowsweet, Peppermint, Chamomile

Herbal Steam: Sinus Steam, Relax Bath

Herbal Bath: Yarrow, Passionflower, Chamomile, Relax Bath

Heating Pad

Indigestion

See Chapter 11: The Role of the Digestive System, page 93.

Simple Infusions: Peppermint, Chamomile, Spearmint

Infusion Recipe: Digest & Rest

Simple Decoctions: Marshmallow root, Ginger, Fennel seed

Decoction Recipes: Smooth Digestion, GI Tonic

Syrups: Ginger

Tinctures: Peppermint, Chamomile

Heating Pad

Nausea

See Chapter 11: The Role of the Digestive System, page 93.

Simple Infusions: Peppermint, Chamomile, Spearmint

Simple Decoctions: Marshmallow root, Ginger, Fennel seed

Decoction Recipes: Smooth Digestion, GI Tonic

Syrups: Ginger

Tinctures: Peppermint, Chamomile

Bath: Catnip, Chamomile, Ginger, Cleansing Bath

Nose/Runny Nose

See Chapter 10: The Role of the Respiratory System, page 63.

Simple Infusions: Mullein, Goldenrod, Catnip, Tulsi, Yarrow, Peppermint

Infusion Recipes: Sinus Clearing Remedy, Breathe Easy

Honey Infusion: Honey/Garlic

Simple Decoctions: Marshmallow, Ginger, Elecampane

Decoction Recipes: Children's Respiratory Blend, Throat Health

Syrups: Elderberry, Ginger, Throat Health

Vinegar: Honey/Apple Cider,

Powders/Capsules/Pills: Cold cap, Yellow pills

Tinctures: Echinacea, Goldenseal, Yarrow

Steam: Thyme, Rosemary, Sinus Steam

Bath: Yarrow, Cleansing Bath

Heating Pad

Humidifier

Pain

See Chapter 12: The Role of the Nervous System, page 101.

Simple Infusions: Boneset (Flu), Chamomile, Peppermint, Catnip,

Skullcap, Valerian, Meadowsweet

Simple Decoctions: Willow bark, Kava

Powders/Capsules: Valerian , Meadowsweet, Turmeric

Tinctures: Valerian, Passionflower, Meadowsweet, Skullcap, Chamomile

Bath: Chamomile, Oats, Relax Bath

Oil: St. John's Wort, Arnica, Cayenne ointment,

Heating Pad

Post Nasal Drip Irritation

See Chapter 10: The Role of the Respiratory System, page 63.

Simple Infusions: Peppermint, Sage, Mullein, Chamomile, Fennel, Hyssop, Spearmint

Infusion Recipes: Post Nasal Drip Infusion, Breathe Easy

Simple Decoctions: Marshmallow root, Fennel , Ginger

Decoction Recipes: Smooth Digestion

Tinctures: Peppermint, Chamomile

Steam: Thyme, Sinus Steam

Heating Pad

Humidifier

Preventatives/First Signs of illness

See Chapter 7: Stages of an Imbalance, page 37.

Food: Bone Broths, Soups

Popsicles: Elderberry

Simple Infusions: Tulsi, Peppermint

Infusion Recipes: Nutritional Everyday Blend, Favorite Preventative Blend, Cheri's Blend, Breathe Easy, Three Lemon Tea

Honey Infusion: Honey Garlic

Simple Decoctions: Marshmallow Root, Elderberry, Ginger

Syrups: Elderberry, Ginger

Vinegar: Apple Cider/Honey Drink,   Winter Root Cider

Powders/Capsules: Green Nutritional Powder, Turmeric, Cold Caps/Yellow pills

Tinctures: Echinacea, Yarrow, Thyme

Steam: Thyme, Sinus Steam

Bath: Yarrow, Cleansing Bath

Heating Pad

Humidifier

Recovery

See Chapter 13: The Role of the Immune System, page 117.

Simple Infusions: Nettles, Oats, Green Tea, Peppermint, Tulsi

Infusion Recipes: Nutritional Tea Blend, Favorite Preventative Blend, Children's Preventative Drink, Three Lemon Tea

Honey Infusion: Honey/Garlic

Decoction Recipes: Energy Root Blend

Syrups: Elderberry, Ginger

Vinegar: Honey/Apple Cider, Winter Root Cider

Herbal Powders/Capsules: Green Nutritional Powder, Liver Tonic,

Herbal Bath: Cleansing Bath, Relax Bath

Humidifier

Sinusitis /Sinus Problems

See Chapter 10: The Role of the Respiratory System, page 63.

Food: Horseradish, Onions, Garlic

Simple Infusions: Mullein, Goldenrod, Peppermint

Infusion Recipes: Sinus Clearing Recipe, Breathe Easy, Children's Respiratory Blend

Honey Infusion: Honey/Garlic

Simple Decoctions: Marshmallow root, Ginger

Decoction Recipes: Children's Respiratory Decoction, Throat Health

Syrups: Elderberry, Ginger, Throat Health

Vinegar: Honey/Apple Cider, Winter Root Cider

Powders/Capsules/Pills: Cold cap, Yellow Pills

Tinctures: Goldenseal, Echinacea

Steam: Thyme, Rosemary, Chamomile, Sinus Steam

Bath: Yarrow, Cleansing Bath

Heating Pad: on forehead and eye area

Poultice: Ginger root on forehead

Humidifier

Sleeping

See Chapter 12: The Role of the Nervous System, page 101.

Simple Infusions: Passionflower, Valerian, Skullcap, California Poppy, Chamomile

Infusion Recipes: Relaxation Blend

Simple Decoctions: Kava

Powders/Capsules: Valerian, Passionflower

Tinctures: Passionflower, Valerian, California Poppy, Skullcap

Bath: Relax Bath

Sore Throat

See Chapter 10: The Role of the Respiratory System, page 63.

Simple Infusions: Peppermint, Sage, Mullein, Chamomile, Lemonade with cayenne powder

Infusion Recipes: Sore Throat Remedy, Breathe Easy,

Honey Infusion: Honey/Garlic

Simple Decoctions: Marshmallow root, Slippery Elm Bark

Decoction Recipes: Throat Health, Children's Respiratory Blend

Syrups: Ginger, Throat Health

Vinegar: Honey/Apple Cider

Powders/Capsule/Pills: Cold caps, Yellow pills

Tinctures: Osha, Sage, Goldenseal, Thyme, Licorice, Myrrh

Gargle: Sage infusion

Steam: Thyme, Sinus Steam

Throat Spray: Adult , Children Throat Spray Recipe

Heating Pad

Humidifier

Throat Congestion

See Chapter 10: The Role of the Respiratory System, page 63.

Simple Infusions: Peppermint, Sage, Mullein

Infusion Recipes: Breathe Easy, Sinus Clearing Remedy

Honey Infusion: Honey/Garlic

Simple Decoctions: Marshmallow root, Licorice, Slippery Elm Bark, Osha

Decoction Recipes: Throat Health

Syrups: Ginger, Throat Health

Vinegar: Honey/Apple Cider

Powders/Capsules: Cold caps, Yellow Pills

Tinctures: Echinacea, Osha, Sage, Goldenseal, Yarrow, Thyme

Steam: Thyme, Sinus Steam

Bath: Yarrow, Cleansing Bath

Gargle: Sage Infusion

Heating Pad

Humidifier

Tonic

See Chapter 17: Be Well, Stay Well, page 245.

Food: Bone Broths, Green Vegetables, Oatmeal, Fermented Vegetables, Kombucha Beverage

Simple Infusions: Nettles, Oats, Green Tea, Tulsi

Infusion Recipes: Nutritional Everyday Blend, Favorite Preventative Blend, Cheri's Blend, Children's Preventative Drink, Three Lemon Tea

Vinegar: Winter Root Cider

Powders/Capsules: Nutritional Powder, Liver Tonic, Endurance powder

Herbal Bath: Beauty Bath

Vomiting

See Chapter 11: The Role of the Digestive System, page 93.

Very small amounts of liquid over period of time. Be careful of drinking too much, too fast, because it will trigger the vomiting reflex.

Chapter 15

RECIPES

I suggest making notes in the space provided on your experiences using herbs and herbal preparations for yourself, your family and friends. For years I kept a 3 ring notebook in which I recorded what herbs and preparations I used and for whom. Herbal Plants work differently for different people. It took some discipline to write my experiences down at the time I was making my herbal remedies but it was well worth it as I used that information time and time again.

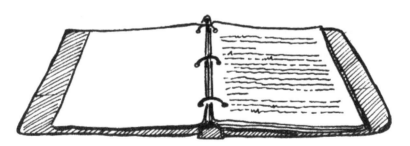

Apple Cider Vinegar/Honey Drink

1 Tbs Apple Cider Vinegar
1 Tbs Honey
1 cup hot water

Combine all ingredients

Bath Recipes:

Cleansing Bath

2 tsp Marshmallow leaf
2 tsp Yarrow
1 tsp Lavender
1 tsp Roses
1 quart boiling water

Directions: Bath

Relax Bath

2 tsp Marshmallow leaf
2 tsp Oats
2 tsp Chamomile
2 tsp Lavender
1 quart boiling water

Directions: Bath

Children's Bath

1 Tbs Catnip
1 Tbs Marshmallow leaf
1 quart boiling water

Directions: Bath

Breathe Easy Remedy

1 tsp Calendula flower
2 tsp Mullein leaf
1 tsp Thyme leaf
2 tsp Peppermint leaf
1 quart boiling water

Directions: Infusion

Calm Cough

1 tsp Marshmallow Root
1 tsp Wild Cherry Bark
2 cups cold water

Directions: Decoction

Cheri's Blend

1 part of Nutritional Everyday Blend Tea
1 part Pomegranate Juice
Several drops of orange flavor oil

*Directions: Make an Infusion.
Cool down and add the rest of the
ingredients. Refrigerate and enjoy.*

*Cheri keeps this blend in her refrigerator
all the time for her family and friends
to enjoy. She makes it in a large
glass container with a spigot for ease
in pouring. A wonderful refreshing
nutritious tea to enjoy everyday.*

143

Children's Preventative Drink

1 tsp Nutritional Everyday Blend
2 tsp Spearmint
¼ tsp Hibiscus flowers
1 tsp Lemon grass
pinch of Stevia (optional)
1 tsp Red Clover blossoms-optional
1 quart of boiling water

Directions: Infusion

Children's Respiratory Blend

1 tsp Marshmallow Root
½ tsp Elecampane
½ tsp Licorice
3 cups cold water

Directions: Decoction

Cold Capsules

1 Tbs Goldenseal powder
1 Tbs Myrrh powder
2 Tbs Marshmallow Root powder
1 Tbs Echinacea Root powder
1 Tbs Ginger powder - Optional
⅛ tsp Cayenne powder - Optional

Directions: Capsules

Cold Sore Infusion and Poultice

1 tsp Lemon Balm
1 tsp Calendula Blossoms
1 cup boiling water

Directions: Infusion or Poultice

Cold Sore Root Blend

1 tsp Marshmallow root
¼ tsp Licorice root
1 cup cold water

Directions: Decoction

Congested Cough Infusion

1 tsp Yarrow
1 tsp Peppermint
1 tsp Catnip
2 cups boiling water

Directions: Infusion

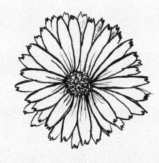

Digest and Rest Infusion

1 tsp Chamomile Flowers
1 tsp Spearmint
1 cup boiling water

Directions: Infusion

Let steep for only 10- 15 minutes.

Longer steeping time results in a bitter tasting tea. The bitterness is very good for the digestive tract but people do not like the bitter flavor.

Dry Cough Remedy

1 tsp Calendula
1 tsp Oats
1 tsp Nettles
1 tsp Red Clover Blossoms
1 Quart of boiling water

Directions: Infusion

Elderberry Juice

2 tsp. Elderberries
2 cups cold water

Directions: Decoction

Endurance Powder

1 part Kelp powder
1 part Nettles powder

Directions: Powder/Capsule
Take with lots of water.

Energy Root Blend

1 tsp Burdock Root
1 tsp Siberian Ginseng
1 tsp Marshmallow Root
1 tsp Sarsaparilla Root
½ tsp Licorice
3 cups cold water

Directions: Decoction

Energy Powder

1 part Marshmallow Root
1 part Siberian Ginseng
½ part Licorice
2 parts Spirilina

Directions: Powder/Capsule

Eye Imbalance Infusion

1 tsp Calendula
1 tsp Mullein
1 tsp Thyme
1 tsp Yarrow
1 Quart boiling water

Directions: Infusion or Poultice

Favorite Preventative Blend

1 tsp Nutritional Everyday Blend
1 tsp Tulsi
2 cups boiling water
1 Tbsp Elder Syrup

Directions: Infusion
Add Elder Syrup to steeped tea.

GI Tonic

1 tsp Marshmallow Root
1 tsp Slippery Elm Root
½ tsp Licorice
3 cups cold water

Directions: Decoction
Strain with large strainer because
this mixture will be very thick.

Green Nutritional Powder

1 part Nettles powder
1 part Oat powder
1 part Alfalfa powder
1 part Beet Root powder
1 part Apple Pectin powder
1 part Kelp powder
2 parts Spirilina powder

Directions: Powder/Capsule

*1 ounce of green powder equals
28 grams or 16 plus teaspoons.*

Healthy Head Tea

2 tsp Wood Betony
1 tsp Nettles
1 tsp Oats
1 tsp Dandelion leaf
1 quart Boiling water

Directions: Infusion

Honey/Garlic Infusion

See Preparation Section

Lemonade

1-2 Tbsp lemon juice
1 tsp honey
1 cup of hot water
Optional: add ¼ tsp. Cayenne
Optional: clove of garlic infused in
¼ cup of boiling water for 10 mins.

Liver Tonic Powder

1 part Milk Thistle Seed powder
1 part Burdock Root powder
1 part Dandelion Root powder

Directions: Powder/Capsule

Nutritional Everyday Blend

2 tsp Nettle
1 tsp Oats
1 tsp Alfalfa
1 tsp Horsetail
½ tsp. Dandelion Leaf
1 quart boiling water

Directions: Infusion

Post Nasal Drip Infusion

1 tsp Peppermint
1 tsp Mullein
1 tsp Sage
1 cup boiling water

Directions: Infusion

Quiet the Cough

1 tsp Marshmallow root
1 tsp Wild Cherry Bark
2 cups cold water

Directions: Decoction

Relaxation Blend

1 tsp Passionflower
1 tsp Oats
1 tsp Lemon Balm
2 cups boiling water

Directions: Infusion

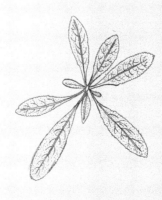

Sinus Clearing Remedy

1 tsp Peppermint leaf
1 tsp Hyssop
2 cups of boiling water

Directions: Infusion

Sinus Steam

2 parts Marshmallow Leaf
1 part Thyme Leaf
1 part Rosemary
1 part Sage
1 Part Calendula Flowers

Combine into a jar.
1 Tbsp per bowl of water

Directions: Steam

Smooth Digestion

1 tsp Marshmallow Root
1 tsp Fennel Seed
2 cups cold water

Directions: Decoction

Sore Throat Remedy

1 tsp Sage
1 tsp Thyme
1 cup boiling water

Directions: Infusion

Sore Throat Tea and Gargle

1 tsp Sage leaf
½ cup boiling water

Directions: Infusion

Sore Throat Hearty Gargle

⅛ tsp Cayenne
½ cup boiling water

Directions: Infusion

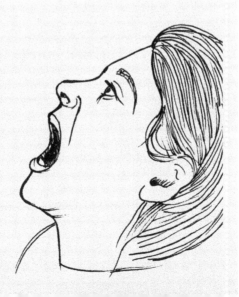

153

Three Lemon Tea

1 tsp Lemon Balm
1 tsp Lemon Grass
1 tsp Lemon Verbena
Pinch of Stevia (optional)
2 cups boiling water

Directions: Infusion

Throat Health

1 tsp Marshmallow Root
½ tsp Osha
½ tsp Licorice
2 cups cold water

Directions: Decoction

Adult Throat Spray

1 tsp Echinacea Tincture
½ tsp Licorice Tincture
¼ cup water

*Combine ingredients and fill spray bottle.
Spray back of throat.*

Children's Throat Spray

1 tsp Licorice root Tincture

1 tsp Honey

¼ cup water

Combine ingredients and fill spray bottle

Throat/Chest Decoction

2 tsp Marshmallow Root

1 tsp Elecampane

½ tsp Oregon Grape Root

½ tsp Licorice

½ tsp Osha root

4 cups cold water

Directions: Decoction

Traditional Gypsy Flu Remedy

1 tsp Boneset

1 tsp Yarrow

1 tsp Peppermint

1 tsp Elder Blossoms

1 tsp Catnip

1 quart boiling water

Directions: Infusion

Uplift

1 tsp. Lemon Balm
1 tsp. Nettles
1 tsp. Oats
1 tsp. Tulsi
1 tsp Peppermint
4 cups water

Directions: Infusion

Winter Root Cider:

See Preparation Section on Vinegar

Yellow Pills

1 Tbs Marshmallow root powdered
1 tsp Goldenseal root
1 tsp Honey
2 tsp Water

Directions: Pills

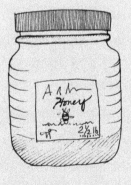

....

Chapter 16
PREPARATION

....

Equipment

Heat proof containers with covers:

Infusions and decoctions preparations need to be covered so the volatile oils of the plants can't escape through the steam; any container that has a top and can withstand the heat of boiling water will work. The herbs should be loose because they steep better in the water than when swished into a metal tea ball. I can't tell you how many people have said that they couldn't make tea with bulk herbs because they didn't have a tea ball. Throw away those metal tea balls: they are useless for making medicinal teas. I use canning jars instead: they are cheap to buy and come in all sizes, and I can always find a lid that fits. Because the lids screw on so tight, they travel well in the car as well.

 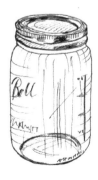 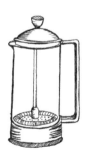

Tea Kettle:

Water should be boiled on a stove. Forget the microwave. Microwave ovens change the molecular structure of food and liquids. Several years ago, a young lady conducted a famous science experiment to prove this: she watered two plants, one with regular water and the other with microwaved water. The microwave plant died 6 weeks into the project, but the other plant thrived. I can taste microwaved water. Believe or not, I am asked all the time how to heat up teas without using a microwave.

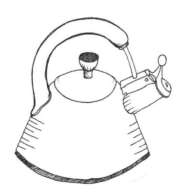

Measuring spoons and measuring cups:

It is important to measure out herbs and liquids when making herbal recipes, regardless of whether or not you're the type of person who likes to make careful measurements. I find that if you measure you don't waste your herbs, and that it is important to measure in order to figure dosages—especially for children.

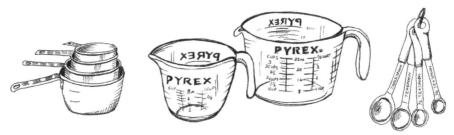

Heat proof glass measuring cups:

I use all sizes of glass measuring cups. I like glass because it is easy to clean. The larger 8 cup glass measuring cup comes in handy when you need to figure out if you have reduced the liquid in half when making syrups.

Strainers:

I use my strainers more than any other equipment in my kitchen. I am always straining infusions or decoctions. For some reason no one has a small strainer in their kitchen anymore. They might have a pasta strainer with big holes, but not the kind of small strainer I'm talking about. I now have to carry one along with my demo stuff when I teach a class since nobody seems to have one. They come in all sizes and with differently sized screens. It is very important to sift herbal powders.

Timers:

I use my timers to time the steeping times of herbal infusions and decoctions.

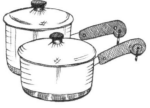

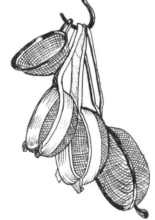

Pots and pans:

Stainless steel or glass pans are fine for making herbal preparations but you absolutely cannot use any aluminum pots. I just use the pots that I cook with on a regular basis. You don't need to have separate pots and pans: this is food.

Knives:

Get good knives and keep them sharp. There's a lot of chopping involved in herbal preparations.

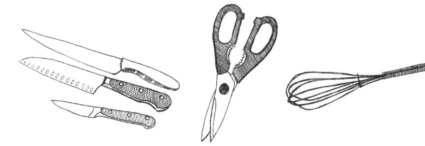

Scissors:

I don't know how I would open anything without my heavy duty kitchen shears. I use them for everything, but they come in handy in particular when chopping up leaves and stems and flowers. Plants are awkward to cut. Use scissors to cut up larger plants into small pieces, then finish cutting with knives. Pruning shears come in handy when stuff is difficult to chop as well. Roots can be especially annoying and difficult.

Wirewhisk:

So useful in blending herbal powders.

Scale:

There are two kinds of scales: regular and digital. Digital scales are inexpensive and work great. Make sure the digital scale can convert from grams to ounces because we live in a society where we need both types of measurements.

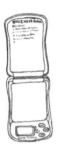 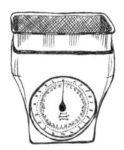 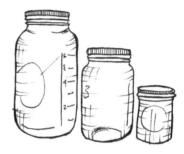

Storage containers:

Glass is the best way to store herbal plants. Again, I use a variety of canning jars, since I can always find a screw top that will work (as the jars are either small mouth or wide mouth sizes).

Labels:

Buy labels from office supply stores and get the type that can stick on plastic bags. If you are in a pinch, use masking tape and a permanent marker. It is essential to label EVERYTHING. Believe me, you will have to throw herbs and herbal mixtures away if you don't get into this habit. I still end up tossing things out because I didn't immediately write out a label: I will make a recipe and not be able to remember what was in it. Keep a roll of masking tape and labels in your kitchen. Never send anything out of your kitchen without a label. Be responsible.

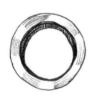 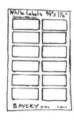 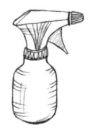 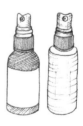

Spray bottles:

There are a variety of spray bottles out there. I have used all different kinds to spray the back of the throat. Most people buy nose spray bottles from the drug store and replace the solution with herbal solution.

Mortar and Pestle:

These are great if you have a small amount of herbs to grind. I have one that has a grooved bottom in the bowl which helps the grinding process. I use mine to grind culinary spices and valerian when I need the powder. A mortar and pestle are easier to wash then a coffee grinder.

Flat River Rocks:

Great for breaking up really hard pieces of roots. I finish off the root pieces in a coffee grinder. I could supply the entire herbal world with river rocks because I live near the headwaters of the Hudson River.

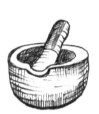 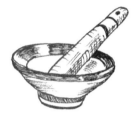 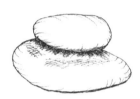

Blenders:

I use my machines to make tinctures and smoothies. I also use it to grind dry plants. The new high power blenders will grind up roots. Tip: The blender blade can screw onto a small mouth Mason jar which is convenient when making smoothies or grinding dried herbs.

Immersion Blender:

I love this little handheld blender. I use it to blend my herb smoothies; it really helps to emulsify the nutritional oil that I use in my shake, which makes it easier on my digestive system. It is much easier to clean than my blender: I just stick it into my cup and blend away. I hate to clean a blender.

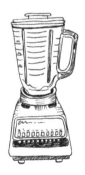 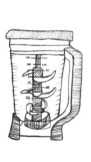 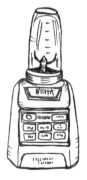 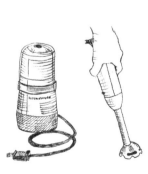

SECTION 2 | *How to Get Well*

Coffee Grinder:

The most-used piece of equipment in my herbal kitchen. I use mine strictly for herbs. Coffee and herb flavors don't mix, so get two grinders if you also want to grind coffee. The new bullet type blenders will grind up herbal plants and even some dried roots. Don't let the grinders get too hot when grinding herbs because you might overheat the herbs: to prevent this, pulse rather than run it for too long. Grinding up roots are the hardest thing to do, so I first crush the hard roots into small pieces before finishing them off in my coffee grinder. Be careful when grinding hard roots, too, because that's how you break grinders.

Capsules:

Capsules come in a wide variety of sizes. I use 00 or 0 size. Personally, I do not like big caps or pills so I like to use the smaller size. When you buy capsule machines, make sure to order the right size.

Capsule Machines:

There is such a thing that will allow you to make a volume of capsules (like my Yellow Caps) ahead of time, and there will be plenty of times when you'll want to have planned ahead for an oncoming illness. Since it just takes two seconds to take a couple of capsules of preventative herbs when coming down with a cold, you will be more likely to help yourself get better than if you need to take the time to brew some tea or, let's face it, lie down and get some much-needed rest. Make your capsules ahead of time with a capsule machine and keep them in your cupboard. Plan ahead. It's like cooking on the weekend for the coming week. Be prepared. The time it takes pays off in the long run.

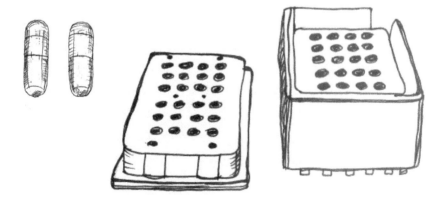

Nylon netting:

I use netting to strain out tinctures and oils and whatever needs to be strained. The nylon netting can be purchased at fabric stores: it comes in different sizes, and the finest mesh is called tulle. A student who made bridal headpieces gave me scraps of tulle once and I have been using it ever since. It's much easier to clean than cheesecloth. I triple the thickness and use it to strain tinctures and herbal oils.

Poultice Cloth:

I keep a supply in my linen closet so I can grab them at moment's notice; you just never know when will need a poultice or compress. I cut up old flannel sheets so I have enough for 100 years. I just send them through the washing machine after I use them.

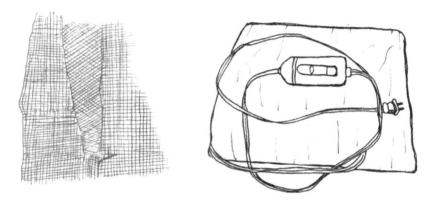

Heating Pads:

There are many different types of heating pads. In the past people used hot water bottles and heating pads. I have several different sizes of microwave heating bags. Please refer to the **Preparation** section for more information.

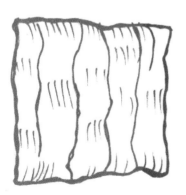
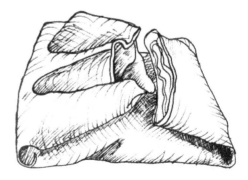

Creating an herbal recipe

When reading an herbal recipe, the term "1 part" is used as opposed to a familiar measurement such as "1 Tablespoon". "1 part" refers to the ratio of the herbs in the recipe. For instance, I use twice as much marshmallow root in my respiratory tea so I would write "2 parts Marshmallow Root" when writing out the recipe for my respiratory tea.

When I first began learning about herbal recipes, I decided to make an herbal tea that would help with my menstrual moodiness and cramps. The recipe I chose contained at least ten ingredients, and the ingredients were listed as "parts". I found an herbal store in Philadelphia that actually carried those particular herbs and would send them via mail order. (Back then, there were no herb stores anywhere.)

I ordered 1 ounce for "1 part" and 2 ounces for "2 parts" and so on. I remember that the bill was very expensive at the time. Still, I was determined to use herbs instead of the drugs commonly prescribed by doctors. I got my herbal package, put all the herbs into a big bowl, mixed it up and made 1 cup of tea. I sat down to enjoy my herbal tea and found that I couldn't stand the taste. (It had licorice in it and at the time I couldn't stand the taste of licorice.) Now I was stuck with a ½ gallon of an herbal formula that I couldn't stand the taste of. That jar of tea stayed in my cupboard for years because I had spent so much money on the herbs; I couldn't bear to throw it away. It just sat there, reminding me to start small next time.

Start Small

I recommend using a teaspoon or tablespoon measurement for your "1 part" when making an herbal recipe. Make a small amount of the recipe, taste it, use it, then mix up larger quantities if you like it. It is possible to buy herbs in bulk in many stores now, so purchase a small amount of the herbs that you are using then create your recipe. **Always, always, always** write down the recipe even if you think you will never forget it. Keep a pad and pencil handy. No need to know why I mentioned this!

Intention

Figure out your intentions for the recipe you're about to make. Is your recipe designed to sedate a cough, or to promote a cough? Be clear about what you want your recipe to achieve, then research the herbs that are "specific" for your intentions. When using herbs that calm down the nervous system, I highly suggest that you stick with one main herb. In our society, it is felt that if one nervine herb is good, four nervine herbs will be better. This is not always so in the world herbal medicinal plants.

Limit your ingredients

I like to limit the herbs of a recipe to three or four plants. If the formula or recipe works and does what it is intended to do, then you will know which herbs are working. When a recipe contains too many herbal plants, it is hard to figure out which plants work and which do not. Sometimes, there is not enough of any herb to make a difference. That is one of the reasons many recipes fail, as there isn't enough of any one important ingredient to make a difference.

Many contemporary herbal books incorporate too many ingredients into their recipes. Their herbal recipes are rarely made because it costs too much to buy all the ingredients for just one recipe (and people think that they have to put every single herb in the recipe in order for it to work). Look at the amount of the individual herbs that are in the recipe.

The herb with the largest amount is probably the one that is most important to achieve the intention of the recipe. Look up that particular herb to see what it does. I once added up the cost of making a cold and flu recipe I saw in a children's herbal book. There were 7 different tinctures and glycerin in the recipe which meant it would cost over a $100.00 to make. Never mind that chances are the children might not like the taste.

Start out with the herbal plants that you know and add herbs for taste and another to compliment the main ingredient.

Traditional Chinese Medicine

Interestingly, Traditional Chinese Medicine (TCM) has produced very complicated formulas that have evolved over many centuries. They never just use one or two herbs; most of their formulas have six to nine ingredients.

Simple

Our herbal traditions are very different. The word "simple" refers to a medicinal plant or it can refer to the tradition of using only 1 or 2 herbs in a recipe. When starting out, it is wise to make your recipes "simple".

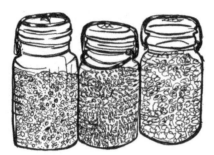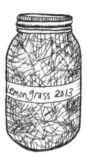

Labeling

My students tell me that I sound like a broken record as I constantly tell them to label their herbs and herbal preparations. I cannot tell you how many herbal recipes I have had to toss in the garbage because I could not remember what was in them. All because I didn't take the time to immediately label them. Jars or bags of dried green herbs look exactly alike. Unless the herbs have a distinctive scent (such as peppermint) or look very different from other herbs (such as chamomile) you cannot tell them apart from each other. Get in the habit of labeling all herbs and herbal preparations as you make them.

Label as you go

Label paper bags with the herbal plant name when you harvest your plants. Label your trays of drying plants. Label your trays of roots. Like dried green herbal plants, roots dry into little hard stones and are impossible to distinguish from each other.

Label your herbs and herbal creations with proper directions

It is of utmost importance that you label herbs and herbal recipes when sharing your creations with family and friends. Verbal communication is all well and good, but once people leave your house they will not remember anything you have said. Don't take my word for this, just ask people to repeat back to you what you've taken the time to explain in detail: they must name the correct herbal plants, explain how they are to be used, and recount preparation

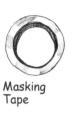

Masking Tape

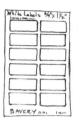

Stickers

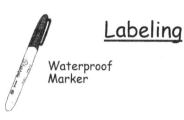

Waterproof Marker

Labeling

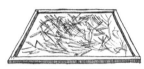

Lemon Grass

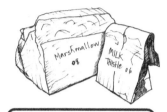

Marshmallow Leaf
Milk Thistle Flowers

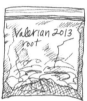

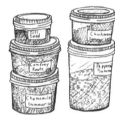

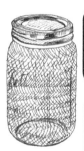

Elderberry Syrup
Elderberry, Honey
1-3 Tbs. daily
Take everyday to prevent colds

Breathe Easy
Infusion: 1 tsp. to 1 cup of boiling water. Let steep for 20 mins.
1-3 cups when needed

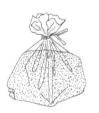

Echinacea Tincture 2017
Echinacea Leaves, Stems, Flowers, Vodka
1/2 to 1 teaspoon when coming down with a cold.

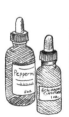
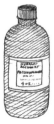

SECTION 2 | *How to Get Well*

directions before they leave your house or office. In most cases, they will only be able to repeat a portion of what you had said. Those well-intended bags and bottles of herbal recipes will sit in their cupboards for years for lack of proper labels and directions.

I send countless jars and plastic baggies to my daughter and son's households, and even though they know what's in the jars they still need everything to be labeled. I once sent a pint of elderberry syrup to my daughter's house and she thought it was tea (either she didn't read the label or I only put the word "elderberry" on the label). She gave the whole jar of syrup to her toddlers. Fortunately, they were fine, but it is important to err on the side of caution.

- List what the mixture is to be used for (e.g. Respiratory Decoction, Flu Tea, Bug Repellent)
- List all ingredients in the bag, bottle, tincture bottle, or oil bottle
- Include preparation directions (e.g. Infusion, Decoction, Syrup)
- Include dosage directions (i.e. 1-2 cups daily, ¼ -½ tsp. daily)
- Record the date the mixture was made.

If the herbal preparation is to be used on the outside of the body (externally), write in capital letters: EXTERNAL USE ONLY. I underline this in red or highlight it with a marker.

Infusion

Infusion is the term herbalists use to describe a tea made from leaves and flowers which is prepared for medicinal purposes. Making an infusion is much like making a regular cup of tea, but you steep an infusion for a longer amount of time and make sure that you cover the container when it steeps. By covering an infusion, you keep all the steam inside the container: if you do not cover it, the volatile oils contained in the steam will evaporate.

Water

As an herbalist I teach about different kinds of herbal preparations, but I always contend that a simple infusion is the most effective preparation. Water is a powerful substance, as we are still learning. Check out Masaru Emoto's *The Hidden Messages in Water*. Water is the most effective menstrum or solvent for dissolving the nutrients in the herbal plants.

Absorption of Nutrients

The body has an easier time absorbing nutrients when delivered via a water-based infusion: it's not about what you eat so much as it is about what your body can assimilate. The body needs to digest and be able to utilize the nutrients contained in an herbal preparation. People take a lot of supplements because there is a perception in this country that we are not getting the nutrients we need through our food. It is hard for the body to absorb the nutrients inside the supplements. Time and time again, people have come to me with digestive problems because their system cannot digest the amount of capsules and pills they consume daily. I believe that a simple, daily tonic infusion made with traditional herbs (like nettles) is all the body needs to fulfill its nutritional needs.

Tisanes

Tisane is the French name for a medicinal herbal tea. As a French Canadian in Maine, my mother remembered drinking tisanes as a child (she would be 90 years old today). She was of the generation that embraced the scientific world of healthcare and ignored the teachings of their mothers and grandmothers, writing them off as old fashioned or not useful. On a trip to France several years ago, she brought me an herbal blend called Tisane des quartes fleurs, or Four Flower Tea. It was a formula that originated hundreds of years ago, made from the flowers of the mullein, malva, coltsfoot, violet, poppy, cudweed, and marshmallow plants. It has endured throughout time and is still being sold as a respiratory herbal tea in Europe. This speaks to the power of plants and their benefits to the world. It brought back many memories of her childhood and renewed her interest in the wisdom of her mother and grandmothers.

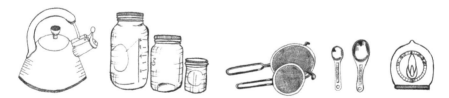

Kettle, Heat Proof Jars, Strainer, Measuring Spoons, Timer

Directions

1. Place the herb or herb mixture into a heat proof container. I use all different sizes of canning jars. I usually make more than 1 cup at a time, so a quart-sized canning jar works well.

Many people ask about little metal herb infusers. They are great in a pinch, but you can't cover the infusion nor allow the herbs to circulate freely if you use one, so it takes too long for the herbs to infuse into the water.

2. Pour boiling water over the herbs and COVER. Covering the infusion while it is steeping is so important because the steam contains many volatile oils: you want to keep them inside the infusion. Let sit for the desired amount of time. (The steeping time can vary from 10 minutes to overnight depending on the strength of the infusion and the different plants.)

3. Strain out the plant material. Use a strainer to strain the plant material from the infusion. After a couple of hours, it is important to remove the spent plant material. Leaving it in the infusion will make the infusion turn. This step is especially important if you plan to make a large amount of the infusion to store in the refrigerator for later consumption.

4. Put the plant material in the compost pile. It makes great compost.

5. Drink the recommended amount of infusion.

Measurement: 1 teaspoon dried herb to 8 oz. or 1 cup of boiling water. Use 4 teaspoons per 1 quart of water. This can vary based on how strong you want the infusion to be.

Dosage: 1-3 cups of infusion daily. If you are taking an infusion for a specific reason, it is suggested to make only what you need for that day (2-3 cups daily). If you are using a daily tonic tea, 1-2 cups is sufficient.

Shelf Life: Tonic teas can be made in quantities and a strained infusion will keep in the refrigerator for several days. You will be able to tell when it is getting too old.

The traditional English therapeutic dose for infusions was usually 1 oz. of dried herb to 1 pint of water. For example, if you were to make a nettle infusion you would use 1 cup of dried nettles to 2 cups of water (M. Grieve, *A Modern Herbal*). If you were to make chamomile tea you would use 1 ⅓ cups of dried chamomile blossoms to 2 cups of water.

It is not necessary to use a large amount of an herb to receive its therapeutic benefits.

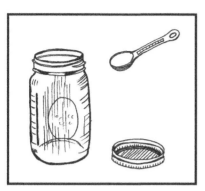

How to make an
Infusion

1. Place herb or herb mixture in heat proof container. 1 teaspoon to 8 oz of water, 4 teaspoons to 1 quart. container. I make several cups at a time.

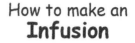

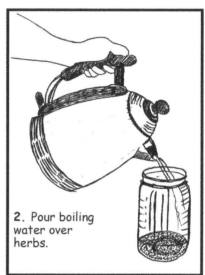

2. Pour boiling water over herbs.

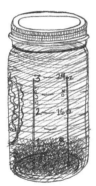

3. Cover and steep for desired time. I steep most teas at least 20 minutes. Nutritional teas I steep till room temperature.

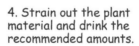

4. Strain out the plant material and drink the recommended amounts.

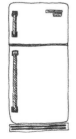

5. Refrigerate the remaining infusion. Do not use a microwave to heat water or to reheat the infusion.

SECTION 2 | *How to Get Well*

Decoction

Decoction is the term for tea made from roots, seeds, or the bark of a plant. Roots, seeds and barks are much denser than leaves and in order to extract their medicinal qualities we need a stronger method of preparation. Plants store the food that they need in their roots for the upcoming year. The roots contain a wide variety of constituents that are different from the leaves of a plant. Decoctions are usually stronger teas than infusions.

I tend to use roots in the wintertime. Many herbal formulas for colds and flu are root-based. I like to add roots to soups for their nutritional and healing properties.

When you dig up a plant for its roots you destroy the plant. Modern herbalists are finding that in the case of many plants traditionally used for their roots, the aerial parts, the leaves, work just as well. By using the aerial alternative, you do not destroy the plant and are able to enjoy the plant's gift season after season. Echinacea is a good example of a plant that was traditionally dug for its roots.

Not only do the leaves and flowers of the Echinacea plant work just as well as the roots, I can enjoy the beauty of my Echinacea plants all season long.

Reusing Roots

You may reuse roots; roots are very dense and can be used several times. The method that works for me is to reuse them immediately. I put half the amount of water in the pan and make another decoction (for instance, if I used 2 cups of water for the first decoction, I now use 1 cup of water for the second). After the second time, I just combine the two decoctions together and drink what I need and refrigerate the rest. If you are using an herbal formula with roots, it is economical to reuse the roots.

Roots and leaves together

Make a decoction. After you have taken it off the heat, place the leaves/flowers into the decoction, cover, and let sit for desired amount of time. Strain and use.

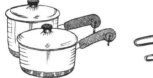 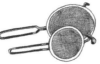

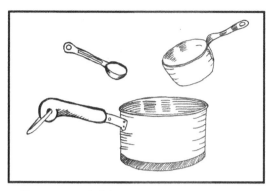

How to make a
Decoction

1. Place roots, seeds or barks into a stainless steel or glass saucepan. Do not use aluminum pans. Put cold water and herbs in the pan.

Measurement: 1 teaspoon to 1 cup of water.

2. COVER

3. Bring to boil, reduce heat and simmer for 20 minutes. I usually make 2 or more cups at a time.

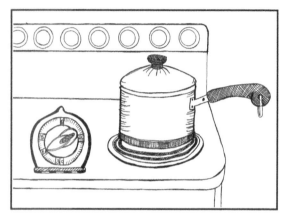

4. Strain out plant material.

Roots can be reused. See directions.

Drink recommended amount.

5. Refrigerate the remaining decoction. Do not use the microwave to reheat.

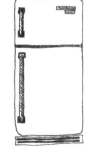

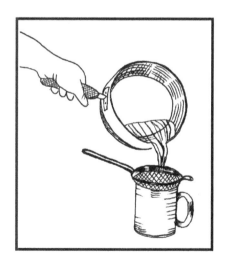

Directions

1. Place the herb or herb mixture in a stainless steel or glass saucepan. Place the appropriate amount of cold water in the pan.

2. COVER the pan.

3. Bring the decoction to a boil, reduce the heat and simmer for 20 minutes. I usually make at least 2 cups at a time.

4. Remove the pan from the stove and **strain** the plant material. For some reason people forget to strain out the herbs from the decoction. The spent herbs will spoil the decoction very quickly if you leave them in. Drink what you want and the rest can be stored in the refrigerator. The strained decoction will keep for several days. You may drink it cold, room temperature or reheat it. Do not use a microwave to reheat it.

Measurements: 1 teaspoon per 1 cup of water. 1 Tbsp. to 3 cups of water.

Dosages: 2-3 cups daily depending on the herb and the sensitivity of the person.

Shelf Life: Keeps several days refrigerated.

Syrups

Syrups are decoctions in which the liquid has been reduced in half and a form of preservative has been added. Honey, maple syrup, sugar are the most common sweet preservatives used in syrups. Roots, seeds, and barks have been traditionally been used to make syrups because they can stand up to the hearty preparation. I have made great nutritional syrups for my children so its good to experiment with different recipes. In the past the ratio of sweetener to herbal mixture was 1:1 but I use a ratio of 1 part of sweetener to 2 part herbal mixture or even less depending on the recipe.

People, children and adults, like to take syrups, which means they "take their medicine". That makes syrups a very effective preparation. Syrups are the way to go when faced with reluctant children or 'sick of the taste' adults. It takes a little more time to prepare but I have found that it is well worth the extra time.

SECTION 2 | *How to Get Well*

Syrups are concentrated so you only need to take a very small amount at a time. Most importantly they taste good and can make a strong herbal recipe taste tolerable. They keep for quite a while in the refrigerator., so they are available to take daily.

I make my very strong respiratory decoction into a syrup as people get tired of drinking the tea. Elderberry makes a wonderful tasting immunity syrup that children love. My favorite is a simple syrup of ginger. Combined with seltzer water it makes a stimulating 'ginger ale'.

Why go to all the bother to make syrups? Because you have a preparation that lasts months in the refrigerator . You only do the prep work once and then have something that you can take everyday for weeks. Again, it taste s good and you only need a tablespoon of herbal syrup. It's a perfect prepara-tion for maintenance doses of tonic syrups.

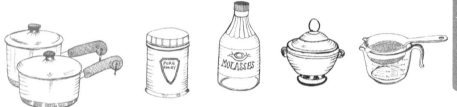

Honey, Molasses, Sugar

Directions

1. Make a decoction. Make at least 2 cups of decoction. You will end up with 1 cup for the syrup.

2. After you have made the decoction remove the lid of the pan (*you may strain out the plant material but I don't*). Let the decoction STEAM not sim-mer. It will start to evaporate slowly at first but it proceeds quickly at the end. It is a good idea to set a timer for 20 minutes and keep checking on the level by pouring the decoction into a heat proof measuring cup through the process. Keep in mind the weight of the plant material. Stay in the kitchen and watch it, I have found that if I leave the kitchen the mixture evaporates away and I am left with a burned pan.

If you are in a hurry pour the mixture into a large bottom pan, the bigger surface the quicker the evaporation process.

3. Strain out the plant material. Now you have 1 cup of double strength decoc-tion. For traditional syrups the ratio was 1 part liquid to 1 part sweetener. That

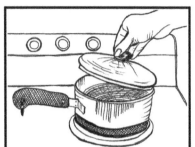

How to make
Syrups

1. Make a decoction. Remove cover and turn up the heat. I leave the plant material in the pan. I make at least 2 cups of decoction.

2. Let the decoction STEAM not simmer until the liquid evaporates in half. It will seem to go slow in the beginning. I set a timer for 20 minutes intervals to remind me. Good idea to stay in the kitchen and watch it. Check on the level by pouring the liquid in a heat proof container throughout the process.

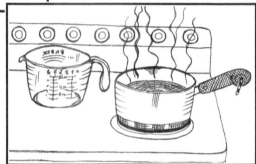

3. Strain out the plant material.

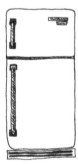

4. Add the sweetener. The traditional ratio was 1:1. I use a 1:2 ratio, for example, I add 1/2 cup of honey to 1 cup of the double strength decoction.

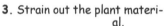

5. Refrigerate the syrup and use 1-2 tablespoon daily.

6. Label your syrup product with ingredients and date.

Elderberry Syrup
Elderberry, Honey
Dec.5, 2017

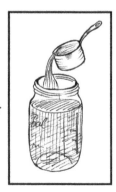

whole point was preserving. I use 1:2 or less. I refrigerate my syrups so I do not need to use so much honey or sugar. The syrups keep well in the refrigerator.

Measurements: Same as decoction, 1 tsp. per 1 cup of water. I usually make 2 cups of decoction which makes 1 cup of syrup.

Dosages: 1-3 Tablespoons daily

Shelf Life: Syrups last several weeks refrigerated.

Herbal Powders

Herbal Powders are easy to make and easy to take. Using herbal powders means that you are taking the whole plant. Capsules are the most popular way to use herbal powders. Capsules are easy to ingest and they travel well. By using freshly ground herbal powders in capsules, you ensure that you will end up with a very effective preparation insofar as it has been freshly made. Herbal powders are also used in pills, and shakes, smoothies, herbal paste (Golden Turmeric Milk recipe) or by itself, combining a teaspoon with a small amount of applesauce.

People tend to use the easiest preparation, which is certainly my way. Filling capsules with herb powders is an easy way to take herbs. I use a nutritional herb powder several times a weeks. I put it into juice along with all kinds of nutritional foods like yogurt, cod liver oil (lemon flavored), and my favorite black cherry concentrate. It might be green but it taste delicious.

I make up my green nutritional powder into capsules so that I will take them every day if I forget to make my smoothie. I also take turmeric in capsules as well. I have to discipline myself to make up my cold cap powder into capsules before the winter cold season begins so that I can grab a couple of ready-made capsules when I am not feeling well. Making your own capsules from your freshly dried and powdered garden herbs is easy and a great way to use your plants.

There is a shelf life to herbal powders. Grinding up the plant exposes it to the process of oxidation, thereby reducing its potency. I grind up enough powder for a month or two's supply and, if I have any powder left, store it in small glass jars in a cool, dark place. You may also store the powders in your freezer.

I had a client who was successfully taking feverfew for migraine headaches. He bought a large bargain bottle of feverfew capsules at a big box store without an expiration date. He started to have migraines again. He never connected the quality and freshness of the feverfew preparation to the fact that the herb stopped helping with his migraine headaches. He purchased some better quality feverfew and was back on track.

Coffee grinders work well grinding leaves and flowers but roots were always a problem. Dried roots are generally hard to grind as they become hard as rocks when dried. I used two large flat river stones that I found in the Hudson River to crush the roots so that I could grind them in my coffee grinder. Some people use a hammer in a cast iron pan. I try to remember to slice my herbal roots into small pieces while they are still fresh.

Until recently grinding up dried roots meant buying a very expensive machine and most people I knew got along fine with other grinding methods. There are now relatively less expensive high powered blending machines that grind up all kinds of things and they work well grinding up herbal roots as well as herbal plants. They make smoothies in an easy to clean container. After 30 years this machine is a welcome addition to my kitchen.

I recommend purchasing herbs that are already powdered if you use a large amount of powders. I order turmeric in powdered form and make capsules as it is expensive to purchase turmeric capsules and pills.

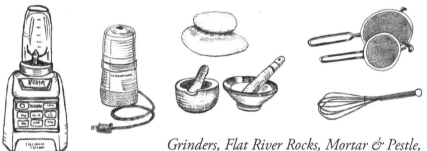

Grinders, Flat River Rocks, Mortar & Pestle,
Strainers, Wirewhisk

Grinding Herbs and Roots

Blenders: Put chopped dry herbs into a coffee grinder or bullet type blender. Grind the herb until it becomes a powder. Grind in short burst to avoid heating up the powder. Grind only enough for your needs at the moment.

Mortar & Pestle: Put a small amount of herb into a mortar and grind the herb with the pestle. I use a mortar and pestle when I need some valerian root for sleeping. I only need to grind up a small amount of powder because

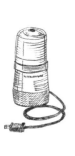
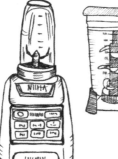
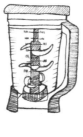

How to Make
Herbal Powders

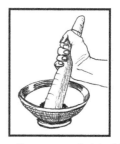

Put dried herb in a grinder and grind till powdered.

Put small amount of dried herbs in the mortar and grind the herbs with the pestle till powdered.

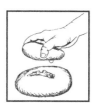
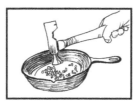

Pound hard to grind root pieces between 2 large rocks or use a hammer and cast iron pan. Finish powdering using a grinder.

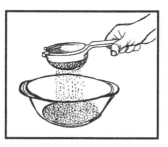

Sift the herb powder with the appropriate size screen strainer to remove larger pieces.

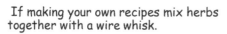

If making your own recipes mix herbs together with a wire whisk.

Store powders in a glass jar in a cool dark place or in the freezer.

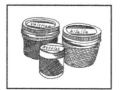

Label your herbs or herb mixtures with the ingredients and date.

Cold Caps
Goldenseal, Marshmallow, myrrh, ginger, cayenne Fall 2016

I usually only need it for a night or so. I keep the valerian roots whole and that way they keep fresh for years. use for small amount of herbs.

River rocks, Hammer and Cast iron pan: Roots that are hard to grind can be crushed by using 2 large flat river stones. Crush the hard pieces of roots into small pieces between the 2 rocks or use a hammer inside a cast iron fry pan. It is important to remember to cut up roots into small pieces before you dry them. I am continuously amazed at how hard small pieces of roots can be, they literally turn rock hard. Finish grinding the crushed roots in the electric grinders.

After grinding herbs it is very important to strain out the larger plant pieces by sifting the herb powder using a mesh strainer. Strainers come in different mesh sizes so pick a mesh that is appropriate. This step is important if you are making pills or shakes/smoothies. You do not want to get a piece of herb stuck in your throat.

A wire whisk works well to blend herbal powders when creating different powder recipes. I make up several different powder recipes every year.

Make sure you label and date your creations.

Measurements: Depending on preparation.

Dosages: ½ to 2 teaspoons per day depending on the herbal mixture.

Shelf life: 1 - 2 year for most powders stored in a dark cool place.

Capsules

Capsules are perhaps the easiest way to ingest herbal powders. In our society, we are trained to take our medicine in pill form which makes capsules a familiar preparation to most people. It is the most popular herbal preparation. Capsules are the way to go for teenagers and people on the go.

My kids grew up using herbs and early on they devised a simple method: Take green caps when you are well, and yellow caps when you are coming down with something. In other words, take tonic Green Nutritional capsules for everyday consumption and the Cold Caps or yellow capsules (which were filled with strong immunity herbs including goldenseal) when sick.

There are many advantages to making your own capsules. Because you are grinding your own herb powder you have control over the *quality* and *freshness* of the powder. It is easy to mix different formulas: by combining different herb powders in certain proportions you can make personal herbal mixtures. It is a great deal cheaper to produce your own capsules as well.

Capsules come in different sizes. The most common are "0" and "00". "0" capsules contain 250 mg (or ⅛ teaspoon) depending on the weight of the herb. "00" contains 500 mg (which equals ¼ teaspoon, again depending on the herb). "00" capsules are large and unsuitable for children. Please inquire about people's size preference ahead of time. You can purchase bags of empty capsules in many stores. They come in several quantities. I buy the 1000 ct.

Gelatin vs. Vegetarian Capsules

There are two kinds of capsules: gelatin and vegetarian. Some people prefer the vegetarian ones because they are made without meat byproducts.

There are two types of machines on the market. "Cap em Quick" and the The "Capsule Machine" They are totally worth buying and using if you want to make your own capsules. Separate the different parts of capsules and load up the machine by pushing the capsule halves into the holes of the machine. I tend to use my " Cap em Quick" machine.

I now have my grandchildren put up the capsules that our families are going to use. We encapsulate the green nutritional powder and the Cold Cap recipe. It is reassuring to have a quantity of capsules in the medicine cabinet when we need them.

  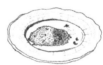 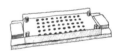

Capsules, Shallow Bowl, Herb Powder, Capsule Machine (optional)

Directions

1. Separate the capsules into the different parts. Put the different halves in separate bowls. (For some reason people love this part of the job. Just ask for help.) When finished, store the unused halves in separate bags for the next time you make capsules.

2. Place the herbal powder in a shallow bowl, maybe ¼ cup or so. Taking the different parts of the capsules in separate hands, scoop up the herb powder into the two halves. I use my fingers to push the powder into the capsule halves.

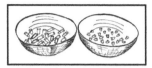

How to make
Capsules

1. Separate the capsules into two pieces. I put the pieces in bowls. Hint: Store the different size capsules halves in separate baggies for next time.

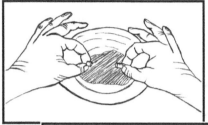

2. Fill swallow bowl with small amount of herb powder.

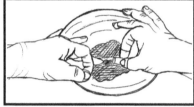

3. Take the capsule pieces in each hand. Start at the distant ends of the bowl and scoop up the powder into the capsule pieces. I use my fingers to push powder into the individual pieces.

4. Push the pieces together.

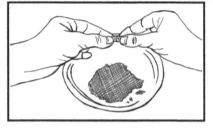

5. Using a capsule machine works very well. I have two different machines. They are time savers.

7. Label with herb and date.

6. Store capsules in glass jars. Store the remainder powder in the freezer or in a cool dark place.

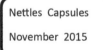

Nettles Capsules

November 2015

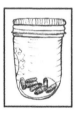

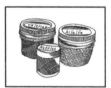
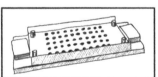
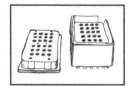

3. Push the capsule together.

4. Store finished capsules in a glass jar.

Dosage: 1-2 "00" capsules three times daily (for the average adult).

Shelf Life: 1 year.

Measuring Powders for Capsules

Herbs are purchased by weight. 1 ounce of dried nettles yields 5+ table-spoons of ground powder. I use about 4-5 teaspoons to make 24 "00" nettles capsules with a capsule machine. According to my calculations, an ounce of nettle powder makes approximately 75 capsules. These volume measurements are similar for other herbs. Herbs differ in weight: for instance, turmeric and kelp are heavier than nettles and alfalfa.

Dosaging with Capsules

Capsules are measured by volume and weight. For instance, a "00" capsule of turmeric weighs 800 milligrams (½ teaspoon). A "00" capsule of nettles weighs 500 milligrams (½ teaspoon). Turmeric is a heavier herb than nettles. So when deciding on the dosage you need, understand that the term *milligrams* refers to the weight of the herb inside the capsules: for instance, if you take 3 "00" capsules of turmeric daily then you are taking 2400 milligrams of turmeric per day. Or if measured by volume: 1 ½ teaspoons daily. There are inexpensive electronic scales that convert grams and ounces that make it easier to figure out what dosage to use.

   Hint: Make sure the capsule maker parts are completely dry before you make capsules. When you rinse the parts the water stays inside the holes for a while. The capsules will melt and the machine will not work (I learned this the hard way when demonstrating with a damp machine for my students.)

Herbal Smoothies

Herbal Shakes or smoothies are terrific ways to take herbal powders. In fact, it has become my favorite way to ingest my daily dose of nutritional herbs. The preparation is as easy as you want it to be. I used to use a blender and blend bananas and all my extra supplements into a "green drink". Then I got tired of washing the blender. (It was a gooey mess.)

My next technique was to use a handheld blender often used to make sauces and soups. It worked great, but then I got even lazier and just put everything in a 1 pint canning jar and shook the whole container as hard as I could. Sometimes the easier the prep the better. Because I try to drink a shake often, I needed to make it a very easy preparation. I leave a month's supply of my green nutritional powder on the counter and pineapple juice in my refrigerator. That way I have no excuse not to drink my shake.

Directions

1. Place 1-2 teaspoons of herb powder into 1 cup of juice. I like pineapple juice, but any kind of juice is fine (my daughter uses pomegranate/blueberry juice for her kids). I have a friend who thinks that tomato juice is the way to go because it holds the herb powder so well.

2. Blend the mixture with a blender or a handheld blender, or by shaking it in a jar with a tight-fitting lid (canning jar lids work well: experiment). Drink immediately. It doesn't keep well.

To make a nutritional herbal shake: Add fruit, nutritional oils, yogurt, fruit concentrates, nutritional yeast, seaweeds (kelp), etc. I like to add 1 tablespoon yogurt, 1 tsp. lemon-flavored cod liver oil, and 1 tsp. black cherry concentrate to 1 teaspoons green nutritional powder recipe in 1 cup of pineapple juice. The shake makes a complete nutritional meal.

Measurements: 1- 3 tsp. of herbal powder to 1 cup of juice depending on your needs.

Dosage: For nutritional needs, 1 tsp. daily

Shelf Life: Drink immediately or within the day.

Labeling: Not necessary.

For I cup of juice I use 1 tsp. of Green Nutritional Powder which contains nettle, alfalfa, oat, beet root, apple pectin, kelp and spirilina powders.

I use 1 tsp. of turmeric paste that I store in the refrigerator, lately I combine turmeric powder with ginger, cinnamon and black pepper.

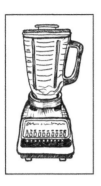

Immersion
Blender

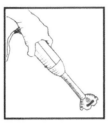

How to Make
Herbal Smoothies

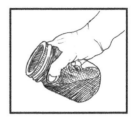

Blend ingredients using a blender, immersion blender or shake by hand.

Herbal Powders
Herbal Paste

Juices: Pineapple, Pomegranate,
Blueberry, Apple, etc.

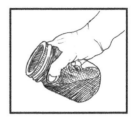

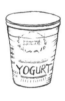 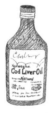 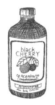

Yogurt
contains
probiotics
or micro
flora

Nutritional
Oils: Cod Liver
Oil, Fish Oil,
etc. Contains
fat soluble
vitamins A & D

Fruit Concen-
trates: Black
Cherry Con-
centrate con-
tains bone
nutrients.

Fruit: Bananas
Blueberries,
Strawberries
etc. contains
nutrients and
bioflavonoids.

Honey is a
ancient
healing
food.

Ground Seeds:
Flax Seeds con-
tain omega 3
nutrients. Milk
Thistle Seeds
contain liver
protective sub-
stances.

Nutritional Yeast
contains complex
B vitamins

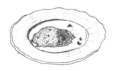

Extra Ingredients

Yogurt: contains digestive flora or probiotics, which are important for digestion.

Cod Liver Oil: contains fat soluble vitamins D and E, and omega 3s.

Black Cherry Concentrate: contains bone nutrients and is a specific for gout and arthritis and joint health.

Honey: an ancient healing food.

Nutritional Yeast: contains complex B vitamins.

Ground Flaxseed: contains omega 3 oils and works as a complex food.

Ground Milk Thistle Seed: contains liver strengthening constituents.

Fruit: bananas, blueberries.

Pills

Pills are easy to make. The basic recipe is to finely grind herbal powders, knead them with a binder herb, cut and roll them into small balls, and then bake them in the oven on very low heat. They can then be stored in a glass jar.

I like to make pills because I like the convenience of taking pills but I don't like to take a lot of capsules. Herbal pills just contain dried herbs. When making pills it is important to use sifted, finely-ground herbal powders.

There are many binders (such as flour) that can work for pills but I prefer to use certain demulcent herbs because they contain gooey substances called mucilaginous that work great for making final products that hold together. I use powdered slippery elm bark or marshmallow root. Both contain healing properties *and* work well as binders.

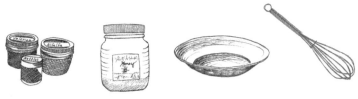

Herbal Powders, Sweetener, Bowl, Whisk

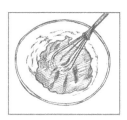

1. Mix the herbal powders Together.

How to Make Herbal Pills

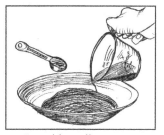

2. Add the binder herbal powder to the herbal powders after the water and honey to create a ball of dough

3. Add small amounts of honey and water

4. Knead the herbal powder till it becomes elastic like bread dough

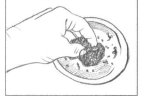

5. Roll out the dough in several long cylinders.

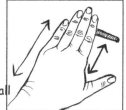

6. Cut roll into small pieces

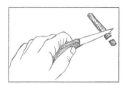

7. Roll out the small pieces with the palm of the hand into small ball shapes.

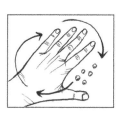

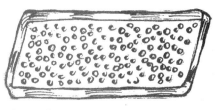

Goldenseal Rt, Marshmallow Rt. Nov. 2017

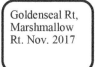

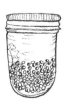

Place pills on baking tray and put in oven on very low heat to dry. Dust the pills with flour or cornstarch after baking.

Store pills in glass jar and label.

SECTION 2 | *How to Get Well*

187

1. Measure out herb powders (except the binder herbs) in a bowl. Stir or whisk til mixed. **It is of the utmost importance that the powders that you use have been strained through a strainer.** Please review making herb powders in the preparation section. You do not want to get any herb pieces stuck in the lining of your throat (which can happen).

2. Put a small amount of water and honey to the herb mixture.

3. Put in your binder herb and knead the mixture until it is elastic like bread dough. Make a big ball. Alternate between the binder herb and water. You do not need that much of the binder herb.

4. Roll out long tubes with your hand. Remember your Playdough days.

5. Cut the tubes into small pieces. **Make them small.** Pills are hard and must be small enough to swallow. This is very important.

6. Roll the small pieces to make them into pill-like balls.

7. Place balls on a cookie sheet and put them in an oven at very low heat till dry, maybe for a couple of hours. You want them to be dry.

8. Sprinkle flour or corn starch so that they don't stick together. Store in a glass jar.

Honey/Garlic Infusion

Honey is a miracle substance. It contains the substances of local wild plants, many of which are medicinal. The bees visit these plants, gather the pollen and turn it into a substance called honey. That is why ingesting a small amount of honey every day is considered to be a type of protection against seasonal allergies. The honey introduces a minute fraction of the plant substances into the body which helps the body build up immunities to the plants that cause allergic symptoms.

Honey contains all kinds of different substances such as protein, minerals, and vitamins. Externally, it is used for all types of skin conditions.

You can use honey internally for cough medicines, sweeteners for herbal preparations (such as syrups), and honey infusions. Honey infusions are time-tested. My favorite is the Honey Garlic Infusion that I make during the cold and flu season.

How to Make Honey Garlic Infusion

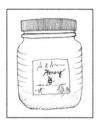

Honey

Garlic

Garlic
Cloves

Jar

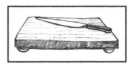

Chopping block

Knife

1. Chop up 6-7 cloves of garlic very fine. I some-times use a garlic press.

2. Place in a small glass-jar. I use a small jelly jar.

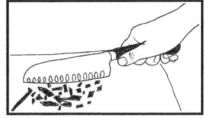

3. Pour honey into jar completely covering the garlic pieces. 1/4 cup of honey will cover the gar-

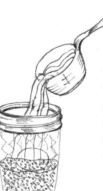

Use several times daily when sick especially in the beginning of an ill-ness. I suggest putting it on a cracker or piece of bread to make it easi-er to take.

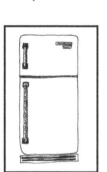

4. Refrigerate the garlic and honey infusion. It keeps in the refrigerator for several months. Label and date the jar.

Honey Garlic
infusion

Jan. 20, 2018

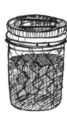

189

Because honey is antimicrobial, it preserves the healing qualities of the herbs in a preparation that keeps for a long time. Because it is sweet, it is an easy preparation to take. I store my honey infusions in the refrigerator where they keep several months.

I always keep a jar of Honey Garlic Infusion and Elderberry Syrup (also made with honey) in my refrigerator during the winter months.

Although there are many herbal preparations available today, that was not the case during most of the years I spent answering panicked questions about what to take when coming down with a cold or the flu. A Honey/Garlic Infusion was a simple solution, and the ingredients were available at any supermarket.

It is still my go-to cold medicine. I recently had an ear problem and the first thing I did was take a ½ tsp of Honey/Garlic Infusion twice a day. It was hard going though, so I suggest using crackers or bread to help get it down. In the past, I would eat a spoonful straight from the jar with no problems.

Honey is so important to me that I put it in my Plant Biography Section. I buy the best local honey I can find. I make sure I stock up every fall. There are dedicated beekeepers all over the North and I make it a point to support their work by buying their honey.

My sister-in-law is a nurse and recently told me that her visiting nurses use Manuka honey, which comes from New Zealand for wound healing.

It is amazing to me to see the quick turnaround of attitudes towards honey and herbs in recent years.

Vinegar Extracts

Vinegar is basically "sour wine". It is made from any kind of fruit or any plant that contains sugar. The action of the harmless microorganisms of yeast turns the sugars of the plant into alcohol; the second fermentation process turns the alcohol into acetic acid to produce vinegar. Vinegar has a history of being used for food and medicinal purposes for millennia.

There are several types of vinegars: Apple Cider Vinegar, White Vinegar, Wine Vinegar, Rice Vinegar and Balsamic Vinegar are just a few. Apple cider vinegar contains many important nutrients: by combining it with herbs and other plants you can create a nutritious food addition. My friend who is a holistic veterinarian says that horses will gladly take their rations in apple cider vinegar. Vinegar is a good preservative and has a shelf life of several years.

The very popular book *Folk Medicine* by D.C. Jarvis, M.D popularized the use of apple cider vinegar as a food supplement and medicine for all types of conditions, for animals as well as humans. He was a Vermont doctor who practiced in the early part of the 1900s. He writes about his experience incorporating Vermont folk medicine methods that he learned from local farmers into his healing practice. He also writes extensively about the healing properties of honey.

My students and I have been making a winter root vinegar for over 20 years. I learned the recipe called fire cider from my apprenticeship program with herbalist Rosemary Gladstar. It is a great winter tonic that some people crave. My students use it as a salad dressing, but people use it for all sorts of conditions. I am not a big vinegar person, but many people do well by adding vinegars to their diet.

Vinegar of the Four Thieves

There are many variations of the origins of the recipe and story of the Four Thieves Vinegar. During the time of the plague in Marseilles, four people would rob the homes and graves of the dead and dying victims of the plague.

When apprehended by the authorities, it was found that they would douse themselves with herbal vinegar in order to deter the terrible disease that was killing so many people. They revealed their secret recipe to prevent being hanged. They were hanged anyway.

FreeFireCider.com

Vinegar recipes are not without controversy in our modern times. For years there has been a lawsuit concerning the name "Fire Cider". Several years ago a company from Pittsfield, Massachusetts trademarked the name "Fire Cider" a recipe that Rosemary Gladstar has freely shared with her students since the 1970's. They proceeded to sue several herbalists who had been using that name for their products. This was very concerning to many of my herbal students. Check out the website for more information about trademarks and traditional products.

This is my version of the trademarked vinegar that I have made with my students every fall since the early 1990s.

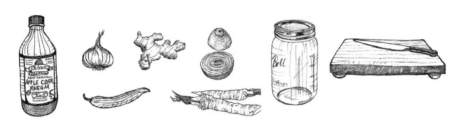

Apple Cider Vinegar, Garlic, Ginger, Onion, Cayenne,
Horseradish Root, Jar, Chopping Board, Knife

1 Quart Canning Jar

Apple cider vinegar (enough to fill jar)

1 large onion peeled and chopped

5 inch piece of fresh horseradish peeled and chopped
(Careful: Fresh horseradish is very strong)

3 or 4 inch piece of ginger, peeled and chopped. (Peel with a spoon.)

1 garlic bulb, peeled and chopped

½ Cayenne pepper chopped, or cayenne powder (optional). (I add cayenne powder after it has steeped as I don't like it too hot.)

2-3 Tbsp. honey

Directions:

1. Combine all ingredients in the jar (except honey and cayenne powder) and pour apple cider vinegar over them.

2. Cover and let steep for 4-6 weeks.

3. Remove the herbs from the vinegar. Pour vinegar back into jar.

4. Add cayenne powder if you have not added a cayenne pepper yet. This step is optional; knock yourself out.

5. Add 2-3 tablespoons of honey. The honey takes a while to dissolve in the vinegar so keep on stirring it in.

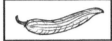 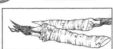

How to Make Winter Root Herbal Vinegar

1. Peel and coarsely chop up the onions, garlic, ginger root and horseradish root. Add a small amount of cayenne pepper if using it fresh. Hint: peel the ginger root with a spoon.

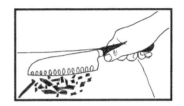

2. Put chopped vegetables in a quart jar and cover with Apple Cider Vinegar. Cover

3. Let sit 2 weeks or up to 6 weeks. Shake occasional.

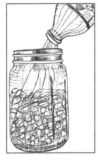

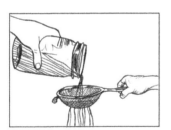

4. Strain out the plants.

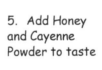

5. Add Honey and Cayenne Powder to taste

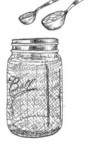

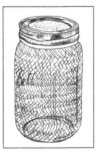

Apple cider vinegar, garlic, onion, horseradish, ginger, cayenne, honey

Fall 2016

Store in glass jar. I put a piece of plastic between the jar and lid as the vinegar will corrode the lid. It will keep indefinitely. Label and date.

6. Put a barrier between the cap and the vinegar. I use a piece of plastic wrap because I use canning lids and the vinegar deteriorates the metal lid after a while.

There are many other varieties of this recipe. I have used burdock root, turmeric root, and different types of peppers.

Four Thieves Vinegar contained the plants of wormwood, meadowsweet, juniper berries, marjoram, sage, cloves, elecampane root, angelica, rosemary, and horehound. But like winter herbal vinegar there are many variations of the Four Thieves recipe as well.

Herbal Tinctures

Tinctures or Extracts are made by combining herbs with a menstruum or a liquid solvent other than water. Although this is a more complicated preparation, more medicine like, it is a useful preparation. The 3 most popular menstruums used in preparing tinctures are alcohol, glycerin or vinegar. The advantages of herbal tinctures are many.

The alcohol, vinegar and glycerin draw different constituents out of the herb than just making a tea with water. For some plants it is a more effective preparation because the medicinal constituents in the plant are not water soluble.

Tinctures last a long time because alcohol, vinegar and glycerin work as preservatives.

They are easy to take.

They are easy to pack. Tinctures dosages are very small compared to teas. They are a great way to preserve a bountiful herb harvest. A great deal of the time, a tincture is the only preparation of a particular herb that you can find.

Making your own tinctures is very easy and has several advantages.

You can combine different plants and make specialized tincture formulas.

The popularity of herbal medicine has made commercial tinctures very expensive, making your own tinctures is a great deal cheaper. If you are taking the tincture for an extended period of time you can go through a 1 ounce bottle very quickly. If you use a quantities of certain herbal tinctures it is wise to grow the plants and make your own tinctures. I make 2 quarts of Echinacea or purple Coneflower every year. It has become a very popular garden plant and it is so easy to make a tincture of the plant, all you need is the plant and some vodka.

U.S Pharmacopeia Standards

The United States has a regulatory agency called the U.S. Pharmacopeia. They are in charge of making sure that our medicines are safe, the quality is pure and consistent, and that preparations are made in a consistent fashion, for example, an Echinacea Tincture made by one manufacturer contains the same percentage of ingredients(alcohol, water, plant) as other manufacturers. Having consistent standards makes it easier to figure out the correct amount or dosage. For example, I take the same amount or dosage from the herbal companies of Herbalist & Alchemist and HerbPharm.

Plants and their constituents are tricky to measure, and measuring the variables is what science tries to do. Plant medicines are particularly hard to measure for consistency. For instance, fresh plants have a high percentage of water, but that varies considerably, think of the leathery leaf of the Rosemary plant in comparison to a the watery leaf of a Comfrey plant. Plants grow in unpredictable environments. They absorb nutrients from the soil but that differs year to year. The soil contains unknown factors each year, their water and nutrient content varies year to year. Some years certain plants do very well and some years they grow poorly. All these variables are hard to measure particularly when making medicines. Science is based on being able to know and measure all the variables. This is difficult when it comes to plant medicine preparations.

When I first started learning about Herbal Medicine in the 1980's, no one concerned themselves with the world of Pharmacopeia. We were just interested in growing and wildcrafting plants and then came the experiments with preparations which were mostly teas. Later as herbalists started different preparations such as tinctures they researched the history of herbal medicine and specially the old Medical and Formula texts in which making plant based medicine is covered extensively.

Southwestern School of Botanical Medicine

The late Michael Moore, a extraordinary herbalist from New Mexico founded the Southwestern School of Botanical Medicine, created a website: swsbm.com which has Fenner's Complete Formulary and Handbook (1888) as well as The Dispensatory of the USA, 20th Edition (1918) and a wealth of other sources for plant recipes and plant preparations for download. In addition he has his herbal handbooks and a amazing amount of information about the contemporary usage of herbs and their preparations. Many of these books that are out of print and are valuable resources about the rich plant traditions and history of plant medicine making in our country.

SECTION 2 | *How to Get Well*

Lloyd Library

The Lloyd library was founded by the 3 Lloyd Brothers in the late 1800's in Cincinnati Ohio. They were pharmacists at the time when plants were the basis of the medicinal preparation in the U.S Dispensatory. Their information on historical herbal usage and herbal preparations along with information on botany, horticultural, and Eclectic doctors is housed at the Lloyd Library and Museum, which is open to the public. Their website is lloydlibrary.org.

Universal Standards

According to James Green in his book "The Herbal Medicine-Maker's Handbook, the standards that were adopted in an intentional conference in Brussels, Belgium, September 1902 ," Conference Internationale pour l"Unification de la Formule de Medicaments Heroiques" are still being used today.

The purpose of this conference was to bring together delegates from other countries and set standards in the preparations of medicines throughout the 'civilized' world. At that time medicine was plant based. They standardized the amounts of water, plant and alcohol in the making of a Tincture preparation so that when one used a tincture preparation from any Pharmacy people would receive a consistent dosage. Tinctures for commercial sale in this country must adhere to these standards. The ratio of plant to alcohol must be stated on the label.

The standards specify the ratio of water, alcohol and plant material when making a tincture preparation which are different when using fresh or dried plants. The ratio for using dried plant material is 1:5 weight/volume and for fresh plant material it is 1:2 weight/volume. The plant material is measured by weighing on a scale and the liquid is measured by volume,(pouring into a measuring cup). Because the average person uses the avoirdupois system of measurement in this country as opposed to the metric system I will use dry ounces for weight and liquid ounces for volume.

For example, you measure out 1 ounce of dried Echinacea root on a weight scale and then combine it with 5 ounces of vodka that you have measured out in a measuring cup. That gives you an approximate ratio of 1:5 weight/volume for your dried plant tincture.

For a fresh plant tincture you weigh out 2 ounces of plant material and then add 4 liquid ounces of alcohol making it a 1:2 weight/volume ratio.

On the label of a 1 ounce bottle of St John's Wort tincture manufactured by the herbal company of Herbalist & Alchemist it states: Dried St. John's wort flower extract 30mL (1:5) in distilled water, 55-65% certified organic ethyl alcohol, St. John's wort flower. This means that they have used the dried St. John's wort plant, ethyl alcohol, distilled water in making this tincture. The Tincture contains 55-65 % alcohol. The 1:5 ratio as discussed above is the standard ratio when using dried plants.

Folk Method of Tincturing

I use these rules or standards as a general guide line. I have been making Herbal Tinctures for over 20 years using a simple but very effective technique. It is sometimes referred to as the Folk Method. I use 100 proof vodka, I let my plants wilt overnight to reduce the water content, and I let the tinctures steep for 6 weeks. This method has worked for me, my fellow herbalists and my students.

Alcohol for Tincture making

The alcohol used in the U.S. Pharmacopeia preparations is 190 proof alcohol. The proof refers to how much alcohol as opposed to water is in the liquid. The higher the percentage of alcohol the better job it does in extracting the plant constituents that are soluble in alcohol. This along with using freshly dried plants makes Tincture preparations more consistent.

In New York State until recently it was hard to find any liquor over 100 proof. So I have always used 100 proof vodka for my tinctures. 100 proof vodka means it contains 50% alcohol and 50 % water provides the correct ratio for my needs. 80 proof means that there is 60% water and 40% alcohol in the liquid and 190 proof contains 90% alcohol and 10 % water. The important factor in making tinctures is making sure that there is enough alcohol in the tincture to extract the properties of the plant and to preserve the preparation.

For example, if you use a 60 proof liquor when using fresh Peppermint leaves in making a Peppermint Tincture, you have to consider the water content of the tincture. The fresh leaves contain a high percentage of water and the liquor contains 70% water and 30% alcohol. That tincture will have a very high water to alcohol ratio. Your concern would be that there isn't enough alcohol to act as a preservative as well as absorbing the constituents of the plant.

I also use vodka because it is a clear liquor as opposed to say Brandy which already has been "tinctured" or has constituents all ready in the liquid. Vodka has very little ingredients compared to other alcohols. Throughout the ages people has been using all types of alcohol in preparing plant medicines. The use of wine has been important. I have a bottle of Herbal Liquor that I purchased in the Austrian Alps in a grocery store. The Herbal liquor is called *Gurktaler Alpenkrauter*. The original recipe dates back to 1050 AD. It contains Rosemary, Juniper, Lavender, Chamomile along with the roots, seeds, and fruits of 59 plants. It is used as a "bitters" or digestive aid. Imagine the same recipe being made for over 1000 years. That's plant medicine for you. Worked in the 1000's and it still works in 2000's to help us digest our food.

Water content of Plants

Plants are mostly water. Drying the plants ensures that it is easier to figure out the ratio of water to alcohol in making Tinctures. Making Tinctures using fresh plants is trickier because you do not know exactly how much water is in the plants so you cannot be sure of your ratios. I use fresh plants most of the time when making Tinctures. I think they are more powerful. In most cases I let the plants wilt for 1-2 days to evaporate some of the water and then proceed. For years I just used the fresh plants and that was fine.

Distilled Water

When making tinctures with a very high percentage of alcohol such as 190 proof it is necessary to add water at the end of the process to dilute the tincture in order to use it. Herbal companies add distill water. Make sure if you are using a higher proof alcohol that you add water in the final step. Consult one of the many books on Herbal tincturing for an understanding of using different percentages of alcohol.

Echinacea Tincture

I make quarts of Echinacea Tincture each summer. I supply many families throughout the year. I see the Echinacea plant everywhere nowadays as it is a beautiful addition to a flower garden. The medicinal species that grows well here is Echinacea purpurea. I show how to make 2 types of herbal tinctures, one is from the fresh plant and the second is from dried roots which can be purchased. The best species for making root tincture is Echinacea augustifolia.

I use the leaves, stems, and flower buds from the Echinacea plant which I harvest in the first part of the summer season. People use all parts of the plant. I do not find it not necessary to use the roots at all. If I did I would tincture them separately and then combine the tinctures. The ariel part of the plant works very well. I realize it is traditional to use the roots but for me the top part of the plant works just fine.

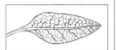

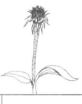

How to Make Echinacea Tincture: Six Weeks Method

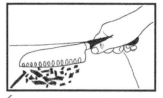

Fresh Plant

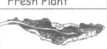

Echinacea flowers

Wilted leaf -left out over night to evaporate the water content.

1. Chop up plant material in very small pieces. Scissors are helpful. I use the leaves, stems and buds of the fresh Echinacea plant.

2. Put chopped up herbs in jar, do not pack it too tight. Leave 1 inch headroom.

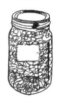

3. Fill to the top with vodka covering herbs.

4. Poke out the air holes with utensil.

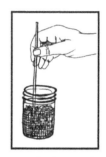

5. Cover with tight fitting cap.

6. First couple of days check to see that liquid is covering the herbs. Add more vodka if necessary.

7. Label jar with date and the date 6 weeks from now. This is helpful in reminding you when to strain out the tincture.

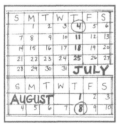

Echinacea stems, flowers, buds, 100 proof vodka

July 4, 2016

August 8, 2016

8. Steep tincture for 4-6 weeks.

9. Shake jars throughout the 6 weeks. Check the level of vodka throughout the process and add more if necessary.

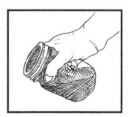

SECTION 2 | *How to Get Well*

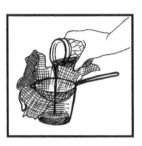

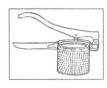

Straining out an Herbal Tincture

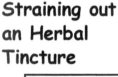

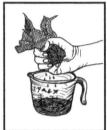

10. Strain the tincture through several thickness of nylon netting.

11. Squeeze with hand or use a potato ricer to get as much tincture out of the herbs.

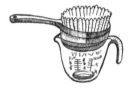

Strain through a coffee filter if desired.

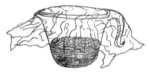

12. Let strained tincture sit over night for material to settle on bottom of container.

13. Pour tincture into storage jars being careful not to pour sludge that has settled on bottom. I fill 1 oz jars for immediate use.

14. Label tincture with herb, vodka, and date. Sometimes I put what garden the plant originated from.

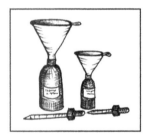

Echinacea Stems, Leaves, Buds, 100 proof Vodka

August 2016

15. Store bottles in a cool dark place.

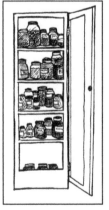

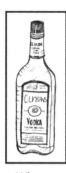

Dried
Roots

Vodka

Scale

Jar

How to Make Echinacea Tincture with Dried Roots

When you make an herbal tincture with dried plant material you use a different proportion of alcohol to the plant ratio. The standard is 1:5 or 1 oz. of herbs to 5 oz. of liquid. They means for, example, if you use 3 ounces of dried echinacea root you use 15 ounces of vodka for the tincture. That is the 1:5 ratio.

1. Measure out 2 or more oz.. of dried echinacea root. I usually use two ounces of Echinacea augustifolia or purpurea root. Figure out the liquid amount that you need. I use 10 ounces of vodka for 2 ounces. 1:5

2. Put both the root and vodka in a jar.

3. Cap it and shake well. Check the levels of vodka for the first few days because the dried root might absorb the liquid, top off with more vodka if necessary.

4. Label tincture with today's date and the date 6 weeks from now.

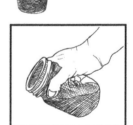

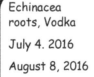

Echinacea
roots, Vodka

July 4. 2016

August 8, 2016

5. Let steep for 4 –6 weeks.

6. Shake jar throughout the six weeks.

201

1. Gather your plant. Let the plant material wilt overnight f desired. It is an optional step. I usually let the large leaves wilt over night. It makes them easier to work with and removes some of the water content.

2. Chop plant material in very fine pieces. Scissors can be very useful in the chopping process. Many herbalists use a blender to chop the plants.

3. Put the plant material in a clean glass jar that has a clean tight fitting top. (Canning jars are very good in this regard because their tops can be screwed on tight.) Pack the plant material in the jar, you want to have enough plant material to fill the jar almost to the top, but do not pack it too tight so that the alcohol can't do its job.

4. Cover the plant material with vodka, using a utensil to poke the air bubbles out of the packed plant material. The plant material should be covered completely. I leave about an inch headroom. The plant material rises to the surface but after a couple of days it settles down.

5. Cover with a clean tight cover.

Check your jars the first couple of days and add more vodka if the plant material is sticking out. Sometimes all you need to do is to stick the pieces under the liquid. I check them during the six weeks as well because sometimes the alcohol evaporates out especially if the cap isn't tight fitting. Just add more vodka.

Sometimes the plants absorb the water in the vodka particularly if they are dehydrated so the jars need to be top off with more vodka.

6. Some people shake their jars during the whole process. It adds a good intention to your plant medicine. I usually forget this part of the process. I leave my jars out on the counter so I will remember what I have tinctured. Some people put their tinctures in the dark. The more attention you pay your medicine the more powerful it will be.

7. Label with the plant name, type of alcohol, date that you have made it and the date when you decant it. I leave the plants tincturing for six weeks. Some people do four weeks.

You can use it any time after two weeks. Sometimes if I need some Echinacea tincture so I help myself to the mascaraing tincture.

I find it is very helpful to put the date that the tincture should be strained out, rebottled and stored properly. I find that decanting the freshly made tincture and rebottling it for the future takes discipline. It is wonderful thing to open a medicine cabinet and have a wide selection of Herbal tinctures all ready for use.

BTW You will not be able to tell what type of tincture it is if it is not labeled. Label it immediately. Just do it now.

8. Remove plant material from the menstrum by pouring the tincture through several thicknesses of nylon netting. Cheesecloth works as well. The hardest part of making tinctures is getting all that precious tincture out of the plant material. I go with a hand squeeze wringing method. Sometimes I use a potato ricer for a better squeeze. If you make a large amount a small wine press works well. They make professional tincture presses. Compost the plant material.

9. Let sit for at least 24 hours for the material that did not get absorbed to settle to the bottom of the container. I use a clear glass container with a pour sprout, I cover it with plastic wrap and I check it every day. I have waited for 5 days for certain tinctures to clear. Sometimes I have doubted that that tincture would clear but it usually does, so be patient. This is an important step in making sure the tinctures have s longer shelf life.

10. Pour the tincture into a storage jar being careful not to pour the sludge on the bottom in the container. If you desired a clearer tincture pour the tincture through a coffee filter. I rarely use this step but sometimes it makes sense. I usually just let the tincture clear up by letting it stand. I use 8 oz. amber bottles for storage and I usually fill several 1 oz bottles with droppers as well. I store my storage bottles of tinctures in a closet in the basement. They keep extremely well in the cool and dark. I store the 1 oz. bottles in my kitchen cabinet.

11. Label your finished product: name of plant, date, sometimes I include the location of when I picked the plant.

Herbal Oils

Herbal oils are easy to make and a rewarding addition to your herbal apothecary. St. John's Wort oil is an amazing healing substance: it helps alleviate painful skin conditions as well as calms down sunburnt skin. St. John's Wort oil has been made for hundreds of years Calendula blossom oil has been used for the health of the skin since antiquity. These striking yellow flowers help cure all types of the "weird skin thingies" that are commonplace in our world.

I learned to make herbal oils by simply cutting up fresh plants and covering them with olive oil and letting them sit for 6 weeks. I had much success. I also had some failures (a very small percentage) when trying this: a few times, mold grew on top of the oils. When I started to teach herbalism I wanted everyone to be successful and not waste good plants and oils, so I introduced some heat methods which produced foolproof oils. Some plants lend themselves to a simple method and some plants are just too juicy and tend to mold in oil, destroying all your hard work.

The directions included in this book apply to two different methods of making herbal oils: a six week method and a gentle heating method on the stove top.

Olive oil
Olive oil is the choice oil for making most medicinal oils. Olive oil has a tradition of being healing unto itself. It is a very stable oil and seldom goes rancid. Until recently you could buy a very small bottle of "sweet oil" for ear problems in the drugstore. Really, it was just olive oil for a hefty price. Using oil for ear problems is a time-honored tradition. Two plants that have a history of helping earaches are garlic and the flowers of the mullein plant. Garlic/Mullein Flower Oil can be purchased but it is easy to make your own.

Garlic Oil
Garlic Oil is made with the cloves of the garlic bulb. It is made on the stove top and can be made quickly when it is needed.

Mullein Flower Oil
Mullein Flower Oil has a history of use for ear imbalances. Harvest the flowers as they appear on the stalk. I collect them until I have ½ cup. Then I use the six week method to make an oil. I combine the garlic oil and the Mullein flower together when I need them, It is not necessary to make a large quantity as you do not need very much oil. It will keep in a cool, dark cupboard for several months.

St John's Wort Oil
St. John's Wort is easy to make. Pick the buds and blossoms after the dew has dried on a sunny day. There is no need to uproot the plant. Usually there are several plants in a field. I use the six week method. I use this oil for many applications. See About the Plants St. John's Wort for more information.

1. Leave herb out overnight to evaporate moisture.

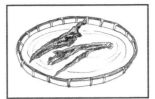

How to Make
Herbal Oils
Six Week Method

2. Chop plant into small pieces. Scissors work well.

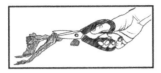
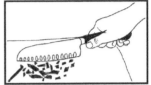

3. Fill small jar 3/4 full with plant material. I like to use 4 oz. canning jelly jars or a small jar. Stay small.

4. Add oil. Oil should be 1-2 inches above the plant material.

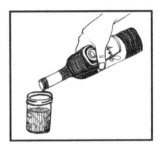

5. Poke out air bubbles.

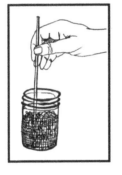

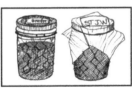

6. Cover jar with lid or papertowel and rubber band.

7. If using a solid cap check the underneath the lid for water droplets during the coming weeks. Wipe the droplets with towel. Make sure there is no plant material above the oil.

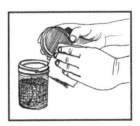

8. Place in a warm spot and let sit undisturbed for 4-6 weeks. It is important to remove the plant material after 4-6 weeks because it will start to mold and ruin the oil.

SECTION 2 | *How to Get Well*

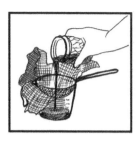

Decanting and Storing Herbal Oils

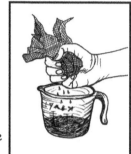

1. Remove plant material by using a strainer lined with several thicknesses of nylon netting.

2. Squeeze out the oil from the plant material.

3. Let oil sit undisturbed for at least 24 hours for the debris to settle at the bottom and the oil to clear. I cover the container with plastic wrap.

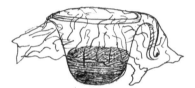

4. Pour the clear oil into a glass jar being very careful to leave the oily sludge into container. Compost sludge.

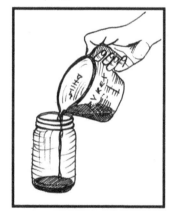

Mullein Flowers, Olive oil
Summer 2018

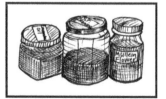

5. Label the jars and store in a cool, dark place. Oils keep for several years.

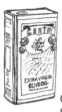

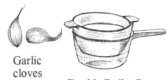

Garlic
cloves

Double Boiler Pan

Olive
Oil

How to make Garlic Oil
Stove Top Method

1. Peel and chop 1 or 2 cloves of garlic.

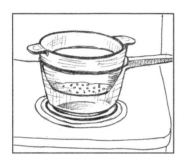

2. Put two Tablespoons of olive oil into the top of a double boiler along with the garlic cloves.

3. Place on stove over low heat for 15 mins. The double boiler pan will prevent the garlic oil from cooking at too hot a temperature.

4. Strain the garlic out of the oil using a strainer and netting. This is very important. Make sure that there are no pieces of garlic in the oil.

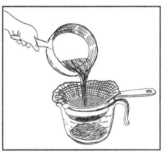

5. Store in refrigerator in a glass container. It will keep several months. Label and date it.

Garlic, Olive oil
Feb. 2017

6. Place several drops of oil in each ear. Warm oil before using it, being careful not to make it too warm. Test it on yourself before using it on a child.

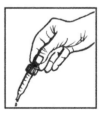

SECTION 2 | *How to Get Well*

207

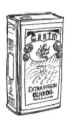 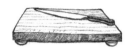 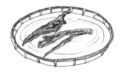

Six Week Method

1. Start with fresh, dry wilted plants. This means that you have picked the plant and have let it dry overnight or for a couple of days to evaporate some of the moisture in the plants.

2. Chop plant material into little pieces.

3. Place plant material in a glass jar. Do not pack the jar too tight.

4. Fill with oil. Poke out any air bubbles with a chop stick. The oil should be 1 to 2 inches over the plant material. If there is any plant material remaining above the oil surface, there will be a greater chance that mold will form on the exposed plants (spoiling the oil). Check jars over the next couple of days as the plant material will float to the surface. Just push it down. One of my students used a plastic screen from a craft store cut to the shape of the jar to weigh down the plant material.

5. Cover the jar with several thickness' worth of paper towels or a coffee filter. Secure with a rubber band or string. You can use a cap, but make sure that the cap is clean and dry.

6. Let the jar sit in the sun for 6 weeks. In the Northeast it is hard to expose the oils to continuous warm conditions. The temperature drops at night, so it is advisable to put the jars in a sunny window rather than outside overnight because the temperature changes are not good for oil. Herbal oils need a constant source of heat to draw out the desired properties. It is important to check your jars, particularly during the first week, to see that the plant material is still covered with oil and to wipe off the moisture that accumulates in the cap. When removing the cap, be very careful not to let the drops of water fall into the oil. Water and moisture will cause the oils to become moldy.

7. Remove the plant material by using a strainer lined with netting; place it into a glass container. Put plastic wrap on the top of the glass container. Let oil sit undisturbed for at least 24 hours. I leave my oils for at least 3 days. Sometimes the oils are very cloudy. I have let oils sit over a week; they become clear. The unwanted particles such as pollen and plant bits settle at the bottom of the container.

8. Pour the oil into another container being very careful to leave the small amount of sludge at the bottom of the oil. Discard the oily sludge. This step will help preserve your herbal oils for a longer period of time. I consider this to be a very important step.

9. Store oils in a dark cool place. They will keep for several years. Light and heat will render them rancid and they will lose their effectiveness. You can smell and taste rancid oils.

Bone Broths

My grandmothers swore by the benefits of many foods that my parents did not. My grandparents were French Canadian. They ate lots of pork fat, real butter, milk with cream on top in glass bottles, and gravy at just about every meal. I remember the big emphasis on gravy and of course the importance of soup. Soup was considered to be healing, especially chicken soup. My grandmothers made soup from bones; my mother opened a can of Campbell's chicken soup when we were sick.

In *Nourishing Broth*, Sally Fallon Morell and Kaayla Daniel not only provide great recipes for bone broth soups but discuss at length the science behind the healing qualities of bone broths. They explain what the broths contain and the particular conditions that are helped by consuming bone broth daily.

Bone broths operate as tonics to the whole body. They contain collagen, cartilage, bone and marrow which help the body repair its connective tissue (including bones, tendons, ligaments, cartilage, skin, hair, and nails).

Long and slow cooking bones releases many healing substances, but the one we are most familiar with is gelatin. That is why cold chicken soup has a jello-like texture. Gelatin has a history of being used as a food supplement for healthy hair and nails. It is commonly added to many food products such as yogurt and ice creams. Collagen is another substance that is considered to be important for the health of bones and joints. As with plant scientists are still discovering substances in broth preparation that contribute to helping the body with such health conditions as arthritis, psoriasis, wound healing, digestive issues and infectious diseases.

Chicken soup is such an age-old tradition for illness that it has been studied by scientists. They have concluded that it contains substances that boost and support the body's immune system which fights off invading viruses that cause colds and the flu.

I have included two easy recipes for bone broths. My family and I consume a lot of soup but broth can be used for many different recipes. All my grandchildren love soup. Right from the time she was a baby, my granddaughter would drink her soup and clamored for more "boff". She only drinks the broth still, and leaves the rest of the vegetables and barley in the bowl.

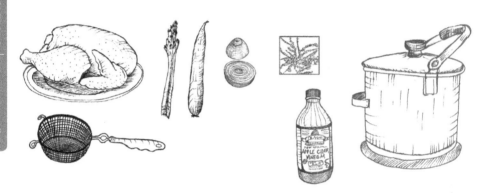

Ingredients for Chicken Broth

Whole chicken (2-4 lbs.) to 2 quarts water.
Gizzards removed.

Vegetables: 1 onion, 1 carrot,
1 celery stalk and other vegetables

Herbs: thyme, parsley,
bay leaves, rosemary

¼ cup apple cider vinegar

Directions:

1. Wash the whole chicken.

2. Place the chicken in a large pot along with the carrot, onion and celery, and herbs such as thyme, rosemary, and a bay leaf.

3. Fill the pot with cold water so that the water level is several inches above the chicken.

4. Cover and bring to a boil. Turn down the heat to simmer and cook the chicken for 1 hour.

5. After one hour, take the pot off the burner and carefully take the chicken out of the pot and place into a bowl. Strip the meat off the chicken carcass and put the skin and bones back into the liquid. Wait for the chicken to cool because it will be very hot.

6. Put the pot back on the stove and add ¼ cup apple cider vinegar to the liquid.

7. Simmer the mixture for at least 2 hours but up 12 hours to create a strong broth. Strain out the bones.

8. There will be a layer of fat on top of the broth. I put the broth in large canning jars and skim off the fat as it rises to the surface. I refrigerate the broth or freeze the broth.

Chicken Soup: Most of the time I make chicken soup immediately. I cook everything separately that I will put in the soup. I like to use barley and small pasta. Barley takes 45 minutes to cook and pasta takes only 10 minutes. I add carrots and beans and, depending on the grandkids, other kinds of vegetables. The cabbage family vegetables are strong tasting so I do not use them for chicken soup. I like adding escarole but it is an acquired taste.

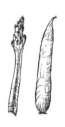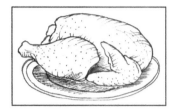

How to Make Chicken Broth

1. Place whole chicken, vegetables, herbs in a large pot.

2. Cover chicken with cold water and bring to a boil. Turn down heat and simmer for 1 hour.

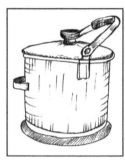

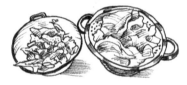

3. Remove chicken from pot and separate the meat from the skin and bones. Place bones and skin back in the pot.

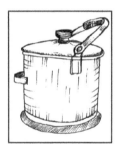

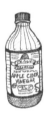

4. Add 1/4 cup Apple Cider Vinegar to the pot and simmer for 2-12 hours.

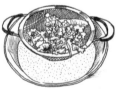

5. Strain out broth from bones and skin.

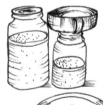

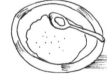

6. Place in containers. I remove the fat when the broth cools and the fat rises to the top of the cooled broth. Refrigerate or freeze. I freeze the broth in cupcake containers and store the individual portions in a freezer bag. I feed my dog bone broth several times a week.

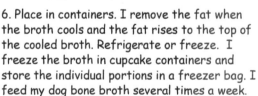

How to Make Beef Broth

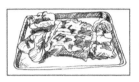

1. Place bones on oiled cookie tray.

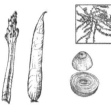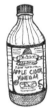

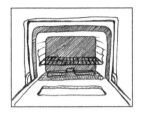

2. Place in oven for 30 mins. @ 350 degrees

3. Put bones, vegetables, and apple cider vinegar in pot. Cover with water and simmer for 6 to 24 hours. Covering the pan is optional. Check the water level during cooking.

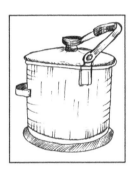

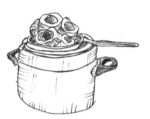

4. Strain out bones from the broth.

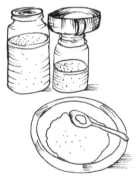

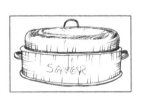

I sometimes use my grandmothers roasting pan for the whole process or a pressure cooker. The new electric pressure cookers work great.

5. Place broth in containers for storage. I remove the fat when the broth cools and the fat rises to the top of the cooled broth. I freeze the broth for later use.

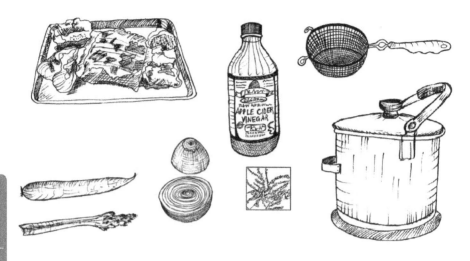

Ingredients for Beef Broth

Bones: I use a combination of different types of bones.
Marrow bones are easy to find:
I combine them with a meaty rib cut.
I use 2 to 3 lbs. for 2 quarts of water.

Vegetables: Onions, carrots and celery
are the staples of making a broth.

Herbs: Thyme, bay leaves, parsley

Apple Cider Vinegar: ¼ cup

Directions:

1. Place bones on a cookie tray (oiled) and bake them in an oven at 350 degrees for 30 minutes til browned. This step is optional.

2. Place the bones and all the drippings in a stock pot and cover it with water. Add ¼ cup of apple cider vinegar.

3. Add vegetables and herbs. I use celery, carrots, onions and herbs such as thyme, parsley and a bay leaf.

4. Place over medium heat, then simmer over low heat for 12 to 24 hours. I cover the pot. Check that the bones are covered with water. Add water if necessary during the cooking.

5. Strain the liquid from the bones. I store the broth in canning jars. I let the fat rise to the top and when the broth is cool I remove the fat.

6. If you freeze the broth in canning jars, only fill them 3/4 full because the broth will expand when frozen. I use strong zip lock bags to freeze broth as well.

Other methods: I use my grandmother's roasting pan to roast the bones. Then I add the water, vegetables and vinegar to the pan while the pan is still in the oven. It is important to check on the water level during this long cooking process. I just turn the oven off when I leave the house or at night, then turn it back on when I am there. Caution: The pan can be very heavy (with all the broth and bones) so I remove the bones with tongs first then pick up the pan when the broth is done.

A pressure cooker works as well. In fact, I use a pressure cooker most of the time now. The new electric pressure cookers that are recently on the market are very easy to use and make a long process much faster.

Golden (Turmeric) Milk

Turmeric Root is the bright orange spice in curry powder. It is a tonic to the whole body but particularly the muscular/skeletal system. In fact, it is one of the best tonic herbs that you can take. It needs to be taken in sufficient quantities in order to be really effective. In India they cook with it on a daily basis. The biggest complaint I have heard is about the taste. Some people cannot get used to the taste. So when my friend introduced me to a traditional preparation called Golden Milk, I knew it should be included in this book. It transforms turmeric into a delicious beverage.

Golden Milk is a two-step process. First you make a paste with water and ground turmeric. You store the paste in the refrigerator. The beauty of this method is that you prepare the paste once and then use it for the next several weeks.

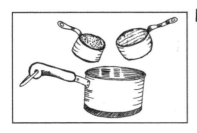

How to make Golden Milk

Making the Turmeric Paste

1. Put 1/4 cup of turmeric powder and 1/2 cup of water in pan. Cook on low heat while stirring constantly. A ratio of 1 part turmeric powder to 2 parts water works well. I cook it for 5 minutes. Remove from the heat.

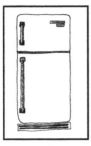

2. Put turmeric paste in glass container and store in the refrigerator. It last for several weeks.

To make a cup of Golden Milk:

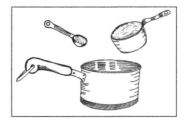

1. Place 1 tsp.—1 Tbsp. of turmeric paste in a cup of milk. Add 1/4 tsp. ground black pepper. Add honey or maple syrup as a sweetener.

2. Heat the milk on low heat till warm. Add spices . I add powdered cinnamon and ginger. If desired add 1 tsp. of a nutritional oil such as ghee, coconut oil, cod liver oil, almond oil, or hemp seed oil.

The combination of turmeric and black pepper is an Ayurvedic tradition .

Black pepper

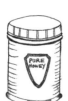

Honey

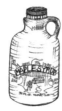

Maple Syrup

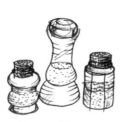

Ginger, Nutmeg, Cinnamon

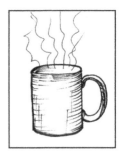

Directions for Turmeric Paste:

Put ¼ cup of turmeric powder and ½ of water into a pan. Cook while stirring constantly. It should take 5 minutes or so.

Put the turmeric paste in a glass container and store in the refrigerator. It keeps for several weeks.

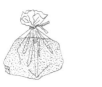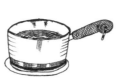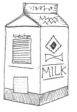

Turmeric Powder, Small Pan, Milk, Glass Container

Directions for Golden Milk:

Heat 1 cup of milk on the stove (no microwave). It can be any type of milk: cow, goat, almond, or coconut. (I stay away from soy milk.)

Add 1 tsp. or more of the turmeric paste along with a sprinkle of black pepper to the warm milk. In the Ayurvedic tradition, black pepper is said to enhance the healing effects of turmeric. It is traditionally added to turmeric preparations.

Add a sweetener such as honey or maple syrup.

Add spices such as ground ginger, cinnamon or other spices.

If desired, add one tsp. of nutritional oil such as ghee, cod liver oil (I use lemon-flavored), almond oil, flaxseed oil, or hemp seed oil.

Drink and Enjoy.

Fermenting Foods

Fermented food is a marriage of salt and fresh vegetables. Combining raw vegetables with a salt water brine for a period of days creates a delicious tasting food but more importantly the fermentation process creates enzymes, vitamins, nutrients and special bacteria that helps our digestive system do its job. Somehow the microorganisms produced by submerging vegetables in a salt brine solution assist the digestive processes. Good digestion is the ticket to good health. Eaten everyday in most cultures fermented foods help the body stay balanced.

Every culture has some type of fermented food that is consumed on a regular basis not just for flavor but for its health benefits. Yogurt is an example of a fermented food which has become extremely popular in the US. The Germans swear by their sauerkraut which is fermented cabbage. Kimchi is a fermented vegetable mixture revered by the Korean culture. I see that all types of fermented vegetables are now being sold at my farmer's market.

Fermented vegetables are called lacto- fermented vegetables because the fermenting process creates a special bacteria(lacto bacillus) which produces lactic acid which in turns preserves and enhances the vegetables.

There are 2 methods of fermenting vegetables: the first method is to soak the vegetables in a salt brine the second method is to sprinkle salt directly on the vegetables drawing out their water to make their own brine. In both methods the vegetables are soaked underneath the brine in an anaerobic process for several days. The most important thing is to keep the vegetables submerged under the brine. The ideal temperature is in the range of 55 –75 degrees. Too hot and the vegetables ferment to quickly, too cold and the process is too slow. Carbon dioxide is produced and expelled. I use a fermenting kit with an airlock which helps prevent unwanted bacteria to get into the fermenting foods.

Sauerkraut is made by salting the cabbage which draws out the liquid making its own prine. Then the cabbage is submerged under the prine for about 4 days. The fermenting process it turns the raw cabbage into a delicious lacto fermented vegetable.

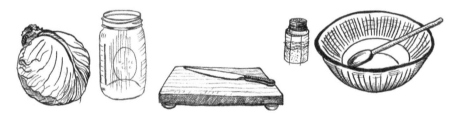

Cabbage, Jar, Chopping Board, Salt, Bowl

Making Sauerkraut

1. Weigh the cabbage. Use the scale at the grocery store produce department. A quart jar needs a 2 ½ lb cabbage. That might seem a lot of cabbage for a quart jar but that is what you will need to fill up the jar after the salting process. Cabbage will vary in weight and size so weighing the cabbage ensures that you are getting the amount you need.

2. Peel off the large outer leaves from the cabbage and save them. Cut out several circles using the canning lid as a template. The leaves are placed on top of the shredded cabbage to help keep the shredded cabbage stay beneath the brine.

3. Slice the cabbage very thin.

4. Place shredded cabbage in a bowl and sprinkle 1 Tbsp. of salt over the cabbage. If you add too much salt the sauerkraut will be too salty tasting. Adding too much salt is a common mistake.

5. With clean hands and a wooden spoon distribute the salt throughout the shredded cabbage. I alternate between pounding the cabbage with the spoon and squishing it between my hands. The cabbage will start to wilt as the salt draws out the water from the leaves. This process takes a while so be patient. Soon there will be enough water or brine pooling at the bottom of the bowl.

6. Pack the cabbage into the jar layer by layer, making sure you eliminate the air bubbles. Leave several inches of headroom. Place the cut out circles of cabbage leaves on top of the shredded cabbage.

7. Put a weight on top of the cabbage leaves making sure the brine is covering the shredded cabbage. It is important to make sure the cabbage is beneath the brine. I use a clay weight but 2 small zip lock bags filled with water will work as a weight for any size of jar.

8. Place a cloth on the top of the jar or fill up the air lock with water and place it on the top of the lid.

9. Label the jar with the date. Place the jar on a plate to catch the excess brine that pushes up through the air lock.

10. After 4 days taste the sauerkraut. If the taste is to your satisfaction you are done. The cabbage will be whiter in color and translucent. The taste will be slightly sour but not vinegary. Eat and enjoy.

11. Put a cover on the jar and store the sauerkraut in refrigerator. It will continue to ferment very slowly in the refrigerator.

Making Sauerkraut

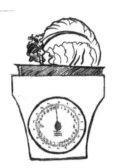

1. Weigh Cabbage : 2 1/2 lbs. for a 1 quart jar

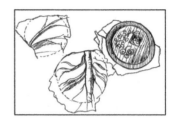

2. Cut cabbage circles from the outer leaves using the top of the canning lid. They are used to keep the cabbage underneath the brine.

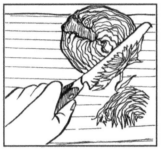

3. Slice cabbage very thin

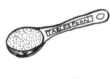

4. Place cabbage in bowl with 1 Tbsp. of salt for 2 1/2 lb. of cabbage.

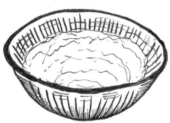

5. Squish cabbage with hands until it is very wilted and the liquid is above the cabbage.

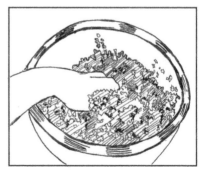

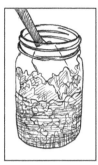

6. Put cabbage into jar packing it down. The brine should be covering the cabbage.

7. Place cabbage leaves over shredded cabbage submerging the cabbage under the brine.

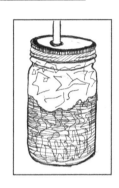

8. Place a weight on top of the cabbage leaves. I use 2 plastic zip lock bags filled with water as a weight . Or there are different types of weights available for purchase.

9. Cover the jar with a cloth or fill the airlock with water and place it in the lid if you are using a fermenting kit.

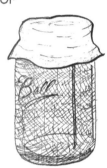

10. Label the jar with the date. Place jar on a plate or tray to catch the overflowing brine

11. Remove the weight and leaves. Cover and store in refrigerator. It keeps for a long time.

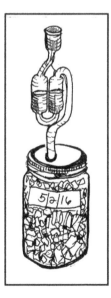

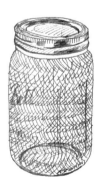

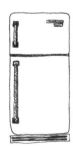

Sinus Steam

Our head contains huge sinus cavities. Bad air, dry air, dust, pollen, and viral, bacterial, and fungal substances can create havoc in our sinuses. Although a Neti Pot is effective in helping to keep some of the nasal passages clear, it does not touch the larger sinus cavities. I found that combining plants that are very high in volatile oils with boiling water and breathing in the steam helps keep the sinuses in working order better than most herbal preparations.

I developed the sinus steam for a young cross country runner who had seasonal allergies and didn't want to use the inhalers he had been using. By steaming in the morning and before he went to bed, the steam cleared the irritating pollen from his sinus cavities; since the pollen was the cause of his allergies, he didn't need his inhalers anymore.

In fact, my steam herbal preparation is my most popular item. Steaming addresses many problems. It is an integral part of moving through respiratory problems such as a cold or flu that affects the sinuses. I steam my sinuses if I feel like I am "coming down with something." It helps several different types of headaches. Up here in the North many people heat with wood stoves, which is a very drying heat: steaming helps keep the sinuses and skin hydrated. Flying affects the sinuses as well and steaming clears the sinuses unlike any other method. Steaming helps resolve a post nasal drip. Besides helping the sinuses, steaming cleans and hydrates the face, too.

Have a box of tissues nearby and blow your nose as you steam. The steam loosens up the mucous in the nose and sinus cavities. In fact, it can help drain congested sinuses.

I recommend steaming several times a day, especially before you retire. I use the same bowl of herbs many times. I put the bowl of herbs into a pan, cover it, and watch until it starts to steam. There is no need to bring the herbs to a boil. Place the mixture into your heat proof bowl and steam again.

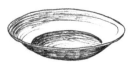 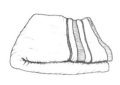 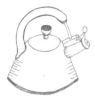

Bowl, Herbs, Large Towel, Kettle

How to Steam Your Sinuses

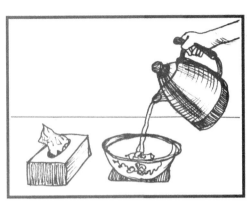

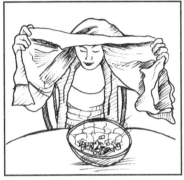

1. Put 1-2 Tablespoons of herbs or herbal mixture into a heat proof bowl. I place a hot pad under bowl.

2. Pour several cups of boiling water over the herb mixture.

3. Cover your torso and head with a large bath towel.

4. Make a tent over the steaming bowl of herbs and steam your face and sinuses for 10 minutes.

Use Common Sense: If the steam is too hot, lift the edges of the towel.

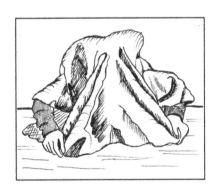

5. Have a box of tissues nearby to blow your nose because the steam looses up the mucous from the nose and sinuses.

The bowl of herbs can be reused. Just cover the bowl until you need it again. Place the mixture in a pan and heat till just steaming. I suggest steaming several times a day.

Plants that work well: Thyme, Rosemary, Sage, Calendula Flowers, Comfrey Leaf, Marshmallow Leaf

1. Place the 1-2 tablespoons of herbs or herb mixture into a heat-proof bowl. I place a pot holder underneath the bowl as it gets very hot.

2. Pour several cups of boiling water into the bowl.

3. Immediately place a large bath towel over your torso and head and make a tent over the bowl. Breathe in the steam for 10 minutes.

4. Use common sense: Lift up the towel if it is too hot underneath the towel.

Caution: Using essential oils to steam the sinuses is recommended in many books. I have found that most people use too high a dosage because it is very hard to measure a small enough dosage (and the oils are highly concentrated). After several days' use, the oils will irritate the sinus cavities as opposed to helping them. If you are using essential oils do not use them "neat" or straight. First, combine them with a carrier oil then add a small amount to your steam.

Poultice, Compress, Plaster

Applying herbal plants directly to the body is a time-honored tradition and what's better is that they work to alleviate all types of conditions. Putting a cut-up onion directly on a bruise will help dissipate the swelling and the black and blue marks. A cooked onion combined with vinegar and flaxseed poultice helps to break the congestion of a cold. A freshly chewed plantain leaf is absolutely the best poultice for bug bites, bee stings, splinters and an assortment of skin problems that we all have encountered.

There are several ways to use herbs in this fashion. A poultice is a combination of fresh herbs or rehydrated herbs wrapped in a thin cloth and applied to the body; a poultice is also the direct application of herbs to the skin using a cloth to keep them in place.

A compress or fomentation is a cloth that has been soaked in herbal tea and applied to the body.

Anatomy of a Poultice and Compress

Dried plants
rehydrated

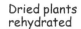

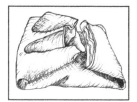

Herbal
infusion

Fresh Plant

Cotton Cloths
for compresses
or poultices

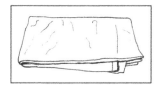

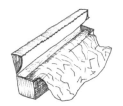

Plastic Wrap is used to prevent
the wet poultices from leaking all
over the place.

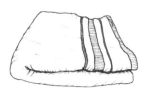

Towel helps keep the poultice
warm and stay in place.

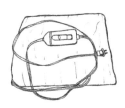

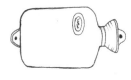

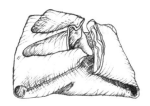

Electric Heating Pad, Hot Water Bottle or Microwave Heat Pads
To keep the poultice warm. This is optional.

SECTION 2 | *How to Get Well*

A plaster is herbs or herbal tea combined with a binding agent such as clay to help the poultice stay in place and add extra drawing power.

Most people have heard of a mustard plaster which is ground mustard seed applied directly to the chest to help alleviate the congestion of a cold. The problem with mustard plasters is their preparation. Mustard seed can burn the skin (as can raw garlic) when applied directly to the skin. Mustard seed needs to be mixed with flour and the plaster must be monitored closely when applied.

A warm or hot poultice has different layers. The first layer is the herbs and cloth or the cloth filled with warm herbs. The next layer is a piece of warm plastic designed to keep the moisture inside the poultice area. The final layer is a towel placed over the plastic wrap, and a heating pad of some type to keep the poultice warm.

For a Poultice on the Go, I use a poultice cloth filled with herbs, plastic wrap on top of the poultice, and wrap the whole thing with stretchy ace bandages to keep it in place.

I learned this when trying to apply a poultice to my ten-year-old son. Of course this works on arms and legs, but I admit that I have used a variation of the Poultice on the Go on my back which didn't work so well. It's hard to sit still and heal. This is not normally an issue when you are sick; the only thing you want to do is to lie down. And that is exactly what you are supposed to do.

Onion poultices are great for so many things and they are great to use for chest congestion. Onion poultices are used to help with bruising, sprains, insect bites, and all sorts of athletic injuries. The compounds in raw onions break up the fluid congestion that results from an injury such as a sprain or bruise. They work as anti-inflammatories: by applying a raw onion poultice to the affected part of the body, the swelling of the wound will reduce to accelerate the healing process.

The book *Ten Essential Herbs* by Lalitha Thomas contains a great chapter on the healing power of onions. In that chapter, she uses her personal experience to explain the medicinal uses of onions, both internally and externally.

A poultice made with cooked onions is a traditional poultice preparation for breaking up chest congestion.

How to make an drawing Onion Poultice for the Chest

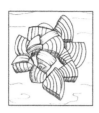

1. Chop any type of onion in small pieces

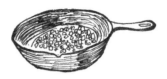

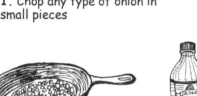

2. Cook onion in pan with small amount of oil on low for 3 to 5 minutes.

3. Add 1 Tablespoon of Apple Cider Vinegar to the onions. This is optional. The smell can be too strong for a child.

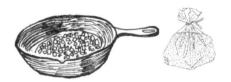

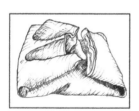

4. Add small amount of Cornmeal or ground flax-seed to make a paste.

5. Place the mixture in a cotton cloth.

6. Place the cloth on the chest. Put plastic wrap over the poultice. Add a towel and then add a heating pad. I use a micro wave heating pad. Leave on chest for at least 15 minutes, checking to see that it is no too warm.

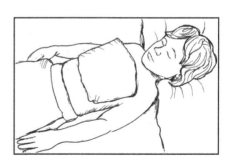

SECTION 2 | *How to Get Well*

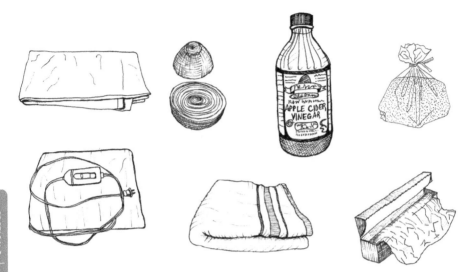

Cotton Cloth, Onion, Apple Cider Vinegar, Ground Flaxseed,
Heating Pad, Towel, Plastic Wrap

Directions:

1. Coarsely chop up a fresh onion.

2. Place the onion in a pan with a small amount of oil and cook it for 3 to 5 minutes. Do not cook it too thoroughly. I just do so until it becomes translucent. Some people do not cook the onion at all.

3. Add a small amount of apple cider vinegar to the cooked onions. This is an optional step. Vinegar has a strong smell which might bother a child. (Although when people are sick they cannot smell because of head congestion.)

4. Add a small amount cornmeal or ground flaxseed meal to the mixture to hold it together. Flaxseed has drawing powers as well. This is optional as well.

5. Place the mixture into a cotton cloth. It will be very warm. Test the temperature before you place the poultice on the chest. Place a piece of plastic wrap around the poultice. Place a towel on top of the plastic wrap and add a heating pad on top of that. Leave the poultice on the chest for 15 minutes or longer. Check the poultice and the chest area.

Bathing/Foot Bath

The first time I tried to use herbs in my bath I just dumped a handful of lavender buds, rose petals, and marshmallow leaves into my hot bath. It was a messy affair: the pieces of plants were stuck all over my wet body when I got out of the tub (never mind the mess when draining the tub). Pieces of plants were everywhere. Fortunately, that is no way to utilize the healing powers of an herbal soak. The best way to make an herbal bath is to make a big pot of an herbal infusion, let it STEEP for at least 30 or so minutes, and then pour the STRAINED tea into a warm bath. Basically, you are soaking in a big cup of herbal tea.

Although I use fragrant rose petals, chamomile flowers, lavender buds and other assorted herbs for a relaxing herbal soak, I find that when I am sick the yarrow plant is a blessing. In fact, I add yarrow to my flower herbal blend when I need a warm and reviving bath (which is often in the winter). Yarrow works as a diaphoretic plant which means that it helps open up the pores in the skin. It makes the body sweat, helping one move the illness out of the body.

1. Select a container to make the infusion. I use a quart jar for a foot bath and a 2 quart jar for a bath. I use several tablespoons for a quart jar and ¼ cup of an herb or herbal mixture for a 2 quart jar. I have also filled up a big pot with water, brought it to a boil, shut off the heat, put a handful of herbs into the pot, and let it sit for at least an hour.

2. Steep for 30 minutes or more (up to several hours).

3. Strain the herbs from the infusion. Be careful when juggling a strainer and a large hot jar. I wrap the infusion jar (which is usually hot) with a dish towel so that I don't burn myself. From years of experience, I have learned that people do not like weird pieces of stuff floating around in their bath so you should make an effort to strain all the herbs out of the infusion before adding it to a bath.

4. Soak in the bath for at least 10 minutes. Be careful when getting in and out of the bath, especially if you do not feel well.

5. A foot bath is much easier to negotiate if you do not feel up to getting in a tub. Many people do not have tubs, only showers, so this is a good solution. Wrap yourself with a blanket to keep warm and soak your feet. They have reflexes that benefit the whole body.

Making an Herbal Bath or Foot

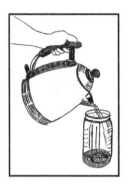

1. Pour boiling water over the herbal mixture . I use a quart jar for a foot bath or a 2 quart jar with for a tub.

2. Cover and let steep for at least 30 minutes.

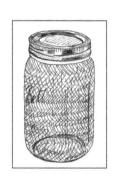

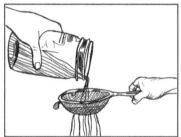

3. Strain out the herbs.

4. Pour the strained mixture into a already prepared hot bath or a into a hot foot bath. Make sure you strain all the herbs out of the infusion before adding to the hot bath.

Soak in tub for 10 minutes or more.

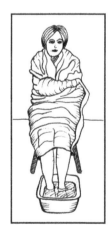

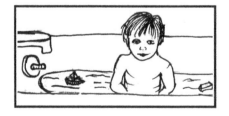

Soak feet for 10 minutes or more

Throat, Nose, Mouth Techniques

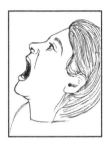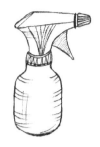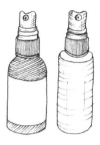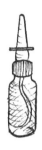

Gargling, sprays, nasal sprays

Gargling works very well to alleviate the pain of a sore throat. I gargle with a sage infusion which is specific for throat problems. Wrap a towel around your neck and gargle away making sure that the tea reaches down the throat.

I also use Echinacea Tincture combined with a small amount of water or tea in a small spray bottle. Echinacea Tincture numbs the throat and helps with throat soreness.

Although I do not use nasal sprays, they are very popular and their containers can be found in most stores. Combining salt water with an herbal infusion preparation can be helpful. Please be very cautious when using essential oils in your nasal solution because they are extremely strong and can irritate the nasal passages.

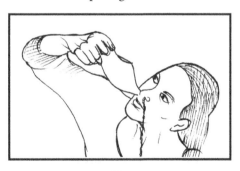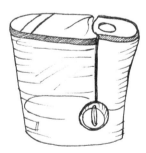

Neti pots are an effective way to prevent an illness because they keep the nasal passages clean and free of germs. Use the salt preparations that dissolve easily in the water. Neti pots are very popular nowadays and are available in many stores.

Warm Air Humidifiers are essential to use when suffering form head and chest congestion. Buy one for every bedroom.

Apply a drop of Licorice Tincture to a cold sore to shrink it and get pain relief. Start as soon as you feel the beginnings of a cold sore. Apply the tincture as much as possible and it will help prevent the sore from getting larger. I put a small amount of tincture in another dropper bottle to prevent the original tincture bottle from becoming contaminated. Sometimes the tincture dropper can touch the cold sore when applying the tincture so this way you prevent contaminating the original bottle.

Eye Wash

Imagine my surprise when I went from drugstore to drugstore in an attempt to find a glass eye cup only to find that nobody carried them anymore! I was looking for a cup for a friend who had acquired the grown-up version of pink eye. I have had great success with herbal eye washes for a variety of eye irritations and had always been able to purchase glass eye cups at any drugstore. They were a drugstore staple not too long ago. Apparently, glass eye cups are considered to be antiques nowadays. Hopefully using an eye wash hasn't been put in that category! My friends said that they used a soup spoon when growing up to bath the eyes. They remember using a boric acid solution which was common for all kinds of eye irritations.

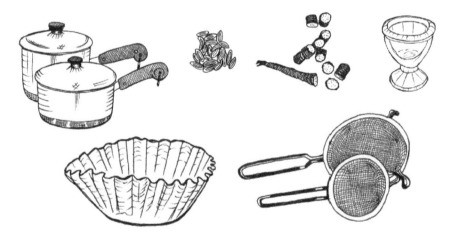

Pan with a Cover, Fennel Seeds, Comfrey Roots,
Eye Cup, Strainer, Coffee Filter

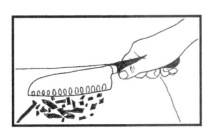

How to Make a Comfrey Root and Fennel Eye Wash

1. Chop up the roots if they are big or fresh. Dried comfrey roots are not too hard to chop.

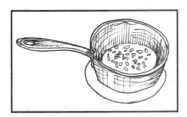

2. Place the comfrey roots and fennel seeds roots in a pan. Bring to a boil and then simmer for 10 mins.

3. Strain out the plant material using a coffee filter. It is important to remove all pieces of plant material from the herbal solution.

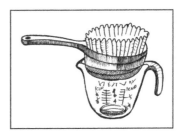

4. Place the solution in the eye cup. Make sure the solution is barely warm so as not to burn your eyes! Test it on your face before you use it!

5. Place the eyecup snugly on the eye socket and let your eye soak. Blink several times to get the solution in the eye. Treat both eyes. Use fresh solution for each eye.

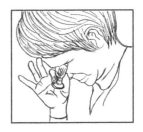

6. Refrigerate the remainder solution. Warm the solution up before using it again. It will keep for several days.

SECTION 2 | *How to Get Well*

Directions for Herbal Eye Wash

1. Make a decoction with Comfrey and Fennel: Place 1 tsp. of comfrey root and fennel seed in a sauce pan. Add ½ cup of water. Bring to a boil and simmer for 10 minutes.

2. Remove from the heat.

3. Strain the herbal mixture through a coffee filter to remove any plant pieces. This is important as you do not want plant pieces in the herbal solution. Cool the mixture down to a comfortable temperature. Always test the temperature on your skin to see if it is barely warm. Again, this is an important step.

4. Fill a clean eye cup with a small amount of herbal solution. I usually fill it almost to the top. Have a towel handy because it can be a little messy.

5. Place the eye cup on your eye socket and let the eye soak in the liquid for several minutes. Blink several times and rotate the eye around. Toss out the used solution.

6. Treat the other eye the same way with fresh solution.

7. Store the herbal solution in the refrigerator and warm it up before using. It is important to warm the solution.

8. Treat each eye several times a day.

Heating and Cooling Pads

Hot water bottles and electric heating pads have been the normative "hot pads" for many years. Microwave bags filled with seeds or grains have become very popular nowadays. They hold heat well and they are easy to use. These bags can also be put in the freezer which can be very soothing for eye strains and headaches. Years ago I heated up kosher salt in a cast iron skillet and filled tube socks with the warm salt for my son's ear aches. Specialty salt has become available: to heat up a bag of salt place it in the oven or toaster oven at 250 degrees for 10 minutes. Another option is bags that can be placed in boiling water or in the freezer which are available at the drug store.

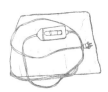 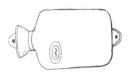

I have received and used many different kinds and sizes of microwavable bags throughout the years. Some hints on making your own:

Favorite sizes: Chest size, 10" x 10"; Neck size, 7 "x 18"; Hand size, 5" x 5"

Material: Use 100% cotton for both the bag and the covering. I use a tightly woven muslin cloth for the bag and a flannel for the cover. I highly recommend making a covering because the bags get dirty from use and they cannot be washed. The covers are easily removed and can be washed.

Filling: Buckwheat seeds, rice, flaxseed, feed corn (NOT popcorn). My experience is that flaxseed is best filling for eye bags that you put in the freezer. Feed corn is good for chest bags because of its weight and heat retention.

Store microwave heating pads in a thick plastic bag. The grains and seeds inside the pads are very tasty to mice. I found this out last winter when I went to get my heating pad from the linen closet at 2 am only to find that a mouse had eaten a large hole in my heating pad, the contents were all over the closet and now all over the floor. Not something you want to deal with in the middle of the night.

Caution: I almost burned down my house on two occasions: (1) when I put dried lavender buds into a flaxseed microwave bag; and (2) when I put the dried lavender buds into homemade candles. Both times the dried plant material caught fire. I left my flaxseed/lavender bag in the microwave at too high a temperature (or for too long) and the oil of the seeds got so hot that it ignited the dried buds, which in turn ignited the cotton material. It was a smelly affair, so unless you are vigilant when it comes to timing don't combine dried plants with seeds. Especially if other people use the bags.

Freezer Bags: Take two small Ziplock bags. Fill one bag with ½ cup of rubbing alcohol and ½ cup of water. Squeeze the air out of the bag and place it into the other bag. Put in freezer. The alcohol prevents the bag from freezing solid and it wraps around the injury or body part better than a piece of ice. The bag can be left in the freezer indefinitely.

SECTION 2 | *How to Get Well*

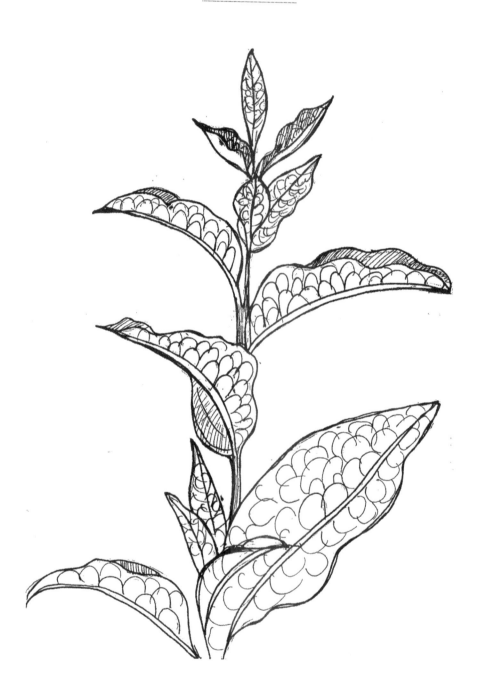

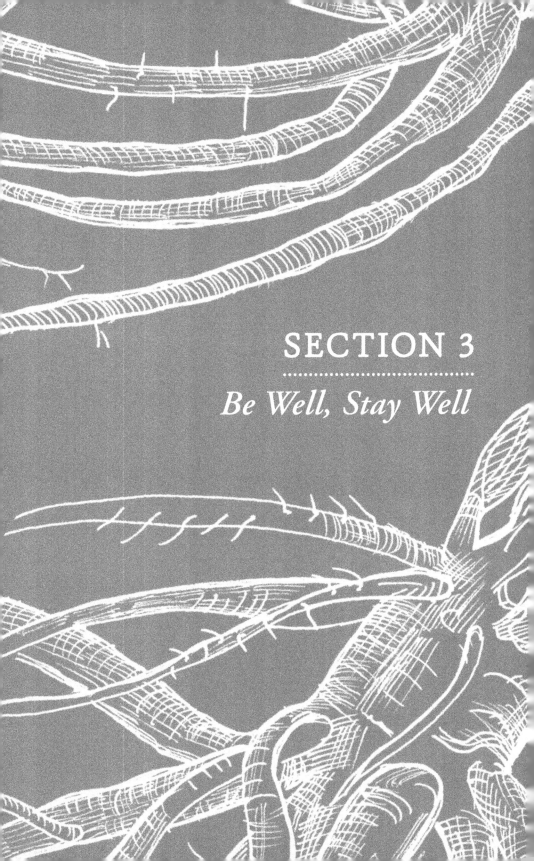

SECTION 3

Be Well, Stay Well

Chapter 17

BE WELL,
STAY WELL

The first step to consider in being well and staying well is our everyday diet. Understand that there is no one diet that works for everybody. But it certainly seems like that would be the case judging from all the constant advice from all corners of the world toting the perfect diet. It is up to all of us, individually, to figured out what are the best foods that work for our bodies.

Are You a Vegetarian? Do you have to be a Vegetarian to use herbs?

I tell people that I eat everything except radishes. Most people I knew when I first started to seriously study about medicinal plants were vegetarians. It was a moral choice as well as a healthy choice. There was a sense in this community that being vegetarian was a healthier and "better" diet. I considered it but I had a husband and kids at home and converting them to an vegetarian diet would not have worked for my family or for I realize me. Years later I heard that several long time vegetarians I knew had health issues that were resolved by adding animal protein to their diets. Today being a vegetarian can means eating fish and chicken everything it seems except for beef. The lines are very blurred. Herbs work no matter what type of diet you consume.

Weston A. Price

In the 1930's a dentist named Weston A. Price was so concerned with the terrible condition of people's teeth in the USA that he set out the four corners of the globe to study traditional cultures (untouched by western civilizations) , what foods they ate and the condition of their teeth. He wrote a book called "Nutrition and Physical Degeneration". It chronicles his travels through the isles of Ireland, Swiss Alps to Eskimos and African communities. He writes in detail about what the traditional foods they consumed and their superb health. He also chronicled the disastrous effect of the western diet of white flour and white sugar to these traditional cultures which was reflected in the health of their teeth and bone structure of their jaws.

When I tried to get this book 25 years ago it was out of print but my local library managed to acquire an original copy from 1939 and I found it to be illuminating. Fortunately it has been reprinted and now is available. There are several organizations such as The Weston A. Price Foundation (www. westonaprice.org) and The Price-Pottenger Nutritional Foundation (ppfn. org) that use Weston A. Price's research. Both of these websites contain wonderful information about nutritional diets. Check out their guide lines on traditional diets, what to eat, what not to eat, the difference in fats and most helpful of all where to buy the food that is being suggested. Weston A Price Foundation publishes a Shopping Guide every year that is very helpful .

Two cookbooks in particular contain recipes and further research on the best nutritional foods to eat and what keeps people healthy. The recipes in "Nourishing Traditions" by Sally Fallon could have been written by my grandmothers. "Nourishing Broths" also by Sally Fallon Morrell and talks about the nutritional power of broths made from bones. Besides the recipes, the research is very compelling on the advantages of making and adding broths to your everyday diet. Again my grandmothers knew all about the power of long simmered soup.

As a child I spent a lot of time in both my grandmother's households. My family is French Canadian and we lived on the coast of Maine. We ate lots of fresh seafood, my grandmothers used butter, the milk was delivered fresh from the farm and placed in box next to the backdoor every day. The cream would rise to the top of the glass milk bottles and I remember my grandmother using it in her morning coffee or tea. My grandfathers both walked to work, came home at noontime for their big dinner and ate a light supper at night. Both my grandmothers were wonderful cooks.

Life with my parents was obviously very different. We never ate butter only margarine, we got our milk in huge plastic gallon containers or sometimes it was made from milk powder which we hated to drink. Both my father and mother worked. My mother did not have the time to cook so we ate lots of TV dinners, prepared box and canned foods and we went out to fast food restaurants frequently. It was a completely different dynamic growing up in both these worlds.

I was the generation of the 50's/60's and we were determined to reinvent the wheel in all sorts of ways. I moved "back to the land", started a huge garden and learned how to cook, can and preserve the food from my enormous garden.

Because of my grandmothers I learned to value fresh ingredients, moderation in eating and because of my French heritage I learned most of all to love to eat and enjoy all aspects of food.

I remember thinking that traveling to a different country meant exploring the local grocery stores as well as the local restaurants along with maybe a museum or two. My mother who travelled extensively would discuss the cultural aspects of a country but nothing would create a level of enthusiasm about a new country as much as the new dishes that she had eaten when visiting.

Buy Local: CSA, Farmer's Markets

People are concerned about where their food comes from and the huge transportation costs involved with getting that food to market. Eating food grown locally makes sense on some many levels. To address that desire for locally grown and local made food and food products look no further than our famers markets.

My area has a Farmer's Market somewhere locally just about every day of the week during the spring, summer, fall and one day in the winter. Community Supported Agricultures (CSA) are all over the country. CSA is a program that a group of people pay a farmer to grow food and then they get a share every week during the growing season. We have many types of CSA's in our area. Essex Farm (www.essexfarmcsa.com) which is up north of me has expanded the meaning of CSA to include all kinds of foods; meat, milk, cheese, vegetables for one price. It has become an extremely successful model of farming. They started in 2003 and have been expanding steadily ever since.

Northeast Organic Farming Association of New York (www.nofany.org) works hard to connect consumers with farmers. They publish a Local Food Guide every year and their web site is filled with information about growing and obtaining local food.

Gardens, Community Gardens

There are several community gardens in my area. They provide people an opportunity to grow vegetables during the growing season. Because of my lack of sun in my back yard I have relocated my vegetable garden to my front yard. It is immensely satisfying to grow vegetables even if it is a tomato plant in a large pot.

The Farm to School Programs

There are several organizations that are dedicated to getting locally grown food to the school lunch programs which are notorious for serving packed process foods. The school lunch program serves food to millions of children across the nation. A shout out to the incredibly hard working individuals of Keene, Schroon Lake and Saranac Lake, New York school districts and others who are serving local food in their lunch programs. October is National Farms to School month. The National farm to school Network helps schools helps schools educate about where the schools hope to promote better dietary choices and help the local farmers. The Keene, New York school district even has a recycling program where they compost all their food waste saving the school district a considerable amount of money. The savings to the school district is considerable, think about the enormous amount of waste is generated by school lunch programs. That waste has to go somewhere and it goes into the landfills at a enormous cost to the taxpayer. To find out about school composting programs go to http://compost.css.cornell.edu/why.html.

Eat a Variety of Foods and a variety of Colors

When choosing food, think of a rainbow and include all colors such as red fruits, lots of green vegetables and make sure you vary the foods themselves in your diet. People get stuck in a diet rut. A variety of different foods provides a large range of vitamins and other nutrients.

Eat According to the Seasons

The supermarket shelves are overflowing with all types of foods from all over the globe no matter what the season. I can get beautiful strawberries at my local supermarket now in the dead of winter. It's 2 degrees outside and those strawberries look so good right now. Spring seems so long ago and it has been a harsh winter. But I will not buy them for many reasons. First of all I do not know where they came from, what type of pesticides they have been sprayed with, and they are not really the type of food that is going to nourish me through this bitterly cold winter. I need something much heartier like chicken soup. The easiest way to figure this out what is in season is to go to a local farmers market and see what is being sold. Greens in the spring and summer, hearty vegetables during the fall and winter.

Cook it Yourself

Learn to cook and make it a fun pursuit. In my years of being a Herbalist I encountered an attitude that **not** cooking was a badge of freedom, almost like cooking had become a symbol of repression. Because these woman did not cook or shop, their dietary choices were very limited, and their health was suffering. When they finally embarked on a wellness program they had to make serious changes in their routines, spending the extra time to shop and cook wholesome meals. Many women choose not to go that extra step and instead wanted a pill or supplement to do that process.

Many young women I know today have no idea how to cook, they never learned at home. I was fortunate in that I learned about cooking for a family from my grandmothers. For them cooking a meal wasn't just putting food on the table, it was how the nurtured their families. They expressed their love through their dinners.

I loved the fact that so many young men I know have taken it upon themselves to learn how to cook. In fact, some of my most enthusiastic customers are young men who have taken the time to learn about the valve of good food and herbs.

Science of Nutrition

The science of nutrition is a relatively new science, the first vitamin was 'discovered' in the 1920's. The science of nutrition studies the processes of digestion, absorption and metabolic interaction, storage and excretion of food. It was discovered that many of the diseases that were common years ago were really vitamin deficiencies. As the understanding of the human body deepens, theories of good nutrition abound.

Nutritional knowledge was confusing when I studied nutrition in college. Nothing has changed in twenty years. It was the best course I ever took for solid information on maintaining the health of the body and I highly recommend taking Nutrition at your local community college if you are interested in any aspect of health care or for your own dietary education. I believe it is a **must** in understanding the human body and its nutritional needs.

However I was amazed at the information I was taught which I felt directly influenced by the agribusiness in our country.

> *Honey is no different than sugar,*
> *they are both just simple carbohydrates.*

No comment about how wrong this is. Honey is a miracle food.

> *Fake fat is fine for the digestive system.*

This was when they were pushing fake fat potato chips.

> *The artificial sweetener aspartame is safe.*

There is so much information on why no one should be using artificial sweeteners.

These questions appeared on the National Test that I had to take at the end of the semester. So it is obvious that one keeps an open mind about the official information from the Food and Nutrition Board (FNB) of the National Academy of Sciences. But with the research capabilities of the internet it is easier to find out who is behind the nutritional information out there such as who is sponsoring the studies. Recently I read that everyone seemed to have a major in nutrition and a minor in food photography.

From my work with people I have noticed several patterns about dietary habits.

Women eat too little protein for their needs and men tend to eat too much.

People do not get eat enough fiber for their digestive needs. My grandmother would have said " Are you eating enough roughage"?

People do not eat according to the seasons, salads are more of a summer food than a winter food.

Too much of prepared foods and fast food restaurant foods are eaten weekly.

They think taking vitamins pills will make up for their poor diets.

Women eat sweets rather than balanced protein foods.

People drink soda and sugar free soda instead of other healthy beverages.

People don't drink water and they don't teach their kids to drink water.

People use coffee as a food instead of eating a nutritious diet. Although they get their energy from the caffeine, sugar and milk in the coffee it's not a good energy source.

Using Tonic Herbs to supplement the diet

There is a huge perception in our country that we do not get the nutrients we need from the food that we eat. People feel that they need to supplement their diets with extra ingredients such as commercial vitamins and all sorts of store bought supplements . The supplement industry is thriving in our country. It is also very hard to negotiate through the maze of what really is good to use for your health and well being. I am often asked about what to take and how much to take of vitamins, minerals and different supplements, although I have studied the science of nutrition I am not trained in for example the use of vitamins as a healing therapy. I use herbal plants to supplement my diet. It seems too simple but drinking a nutritional tea everyday works wonders to supplement the diet with extra nutrients.

In his book "Nutritional Herbology", Mark Pedersen chemically analyses the nutritional profile of hundreds of herbs and foods. When I first saw his l charts I was completely amazed at how high the nutritional content of the herbs that I use particularly the herbs I use on a regular basis. When I show the charts to my students it seems to verify what I am talking about and gives them great comfort to see the measurements of vitamins and minerals all spelled out. If you like measurements seek out this book.

One of the reasons I love herbal plants known as tonics is that they supply the body with the extra nutrients. My favorite category of herbs are the herbs that you can take every day which are loaded with vitamins and minerals

SECTION 3 | *Be Well, Stay Well*

that the body needs to stay and be healthy. The right preparations is also important, you want to get the most value from what you are buying and taking. Know where the herbal plants come from. The fresher the better. Try your hand at growing herbal plants, they don't take up so much room and are power houses of nutrition for their sizes.

Effective Preparations

Several years ago doctors were advising their patients to take mega dosages of calcium to ensure strong bones especially after menopause. Most women were taking large pills of calcium everyday as a health insurance. This all seem to come at the same time that doctor's offices acquired bone densities machines. Today the theory of taking large mega doses of calcium in pill form is no longer in vogue. Keep in mind that Science is based on theory, it changes as new information is discovered.

My biggest selling Herbal product is my Nutritional Blend Tea which is prepared as an infusion. It contains a combination of traditional tonic herbs which are loaded with different nutrients especially with the nutrient of calcium. The combination of herbs is like taking a vitamin pill only better for the body because the body **absorbs** the nutrients through the water based preparation. The nutrients in the herbs are balanced.

Herbal Powders

Another way to ingest everyday nutritional herbs is by themselves, just grind up the dried herbs into a powdered form and put the powder into a smoothie drink , or make capsules. A very simple way to ingest herb powders is to put it into applesauce. It is extremely easy to make herbal powders from dried herbs. Most herbs powder up well by using a simple coffee grinder.

I have encountered all types of nutritional powders that are on the market. My complaint is that they contain a lot of unnecessary fillers such as soy flour and other substances. It is easy to put together your own blend of ground herbs and I used several herbs that I grind myself as well as an algae called Spirulina in my herbal green powder. I blend 1 teaspoon of the powdered herbs with juice, yogurt, Nutritional oil and a banana or blueberries. See Herbal Powders and Herbal Smoothies in the Preparation Section.

My grandchildren all drank "green drinks" as soon as they could drink from a cup. I would see them roving around the house with their sippee cups slurping down their green drink made with juice, bananas and nana's green powder. They would ask for it. This helped my daughter not fret about their vegetable consumption. Getting kids to eats vegetables can be challenging, never mind some adults who refuse to eat them at all.

My Favorite Tonic Herbs

Nettles

There are many herbs that work as tonics to the whole body but Nettles which grows prolifically here, stands out as the most utilized for this reason. Because I live in a rural community there is always someone in my classes who has encountered the stinging nettle plant while walking in a field. It grows in fields and it stings when brushed against because of the formic acid in its leaves. This is the one plant that people that people continue to mis-identify. Half the time they bring me a bull thistle plant because of its thorns or maybe a mature motherwort plant because of its prickles. They have the right idea of the danger of touching this plant. But please when you are first identifying plants go with an expert the first couple of times so that you don't pick the wrong plants.

Oats

I combine the nutritional power of nettles with my other favorite tonic plant Oats. Oats is a grass and is about the easiest plant to grow. Just acquire some seeds throw them into the ground and before you know it you have a stand of oats. Yes this is the same plant they make oatmeal from and we know how healthful oatmeal is. As the plant matures it develops spiklets or mature flow-ers/seeds and when the oats seeds taste milky that is the time to harvest the whole plant and dry it. It is a power house of nutrition.

Tulsi or Holy Basil

One of my new favorite plants is Tulsi or Holy Basil. It is a much beloved plant in India. According to a young Indian lady in one of my herbal classes who sprang to life after tasting the Tulsi tea that was being passed around, people in India drink Tulsi tea in the morning and at night and during the day they go out into the garden pick and eat the leaves of the Holy Basil plant.

I have served Tulsi to hundreds of people and the consensus is that it tastes great. Many people think it is a combination of different plants because of its complex taste. Although it is used for a myriad of conditions I use it as an everyday tonic. Between my family and friends we used this wonderful plant often. See more information about Tulsi in the About the Plants Section. I combine Tulsi with my favorite Nutritional Blend and that is my go to drink for taste and nutrition.

Turmeric

Another gem of a plant from India is Turmeric Root. It is the bright orange spice in curry powder. It is a tonic to the whole body but particularly the muscular/skeletal system. As people get older the wear and tear on their system requires extra care and using turmeric helps maintain a health structure. I have been recommending turmeric for a long time particularly for runners and athelics. The biggest complaint is the taste. Some people can not get used to the taste. So using a capsule or pill preparation would be the way to go. Recently a friend has clued me into a turmeric beverage recipe called Golden Milk. Basically you make a paste of turmeric and water. Store the paste in the refrigerator ; warm up a cup of milk with one teaspoon of turmeric paste, a little honey and a dash of pepper. It is delicious and makes taking turmeric a joy. Check out the Golden Milk recipe in the Preparation section.

Algae

The Algae family includes many different types of algae. The two types of algae that people are familiar with are the cyanobacteria group which includes spirulina and chlorella and seaweeds such as kelp and bladderwort. This group of plants have been used for thousands of years as food and food supplements. Ryan Drum an herbalist from Washington state has been harvesting and using seaweeds for over 30 years. His website (www.ryandrum.com) contains great information about all things algae.

Closer to home is Maine Coast Sea Vegetables (www.seaveg.com) and Ironbound Island (www.ironbound.com) companies that harvest seaweed from the coast of Maine. I use their different types of seaweed in all types of dishes. I throw in a large piece of kelp when making a pot of beans and it makes the beans more digestible and taste better. The Maine Coast website is crammed with the latest on using and harvesting sea weed. It has become a important industry.

I personally use Spirulina, an algae, in my nutritional green powder along with several ground herbs. Cultivated Spirulina has a long history of use. It was used as a food source by the ancient Aztec and Mayan cultures. It is harvested for food from Lake Chad by the Kanembu tribe who reside in the Sahara desert. There is much research done in Japan on the genus Spirulina where they used it as a food and medicine.

Seaweed

Having grown up on the coast of Maine the smell of seaweed seems like home to me. I use kelp in my green nutritional powder along with the spirulina. Originally my green powder contained only kelp and nettles. My kids called it the "green pills' that you took when you were well. I developed it for my daughter who was a long distance runner. We tried many blends of herbs and seeds and this simple combination seemed to work the best. She took it before races and it gave her energy through her race. My take on how it works is that it replaces the electrolytes that are being used up while doing strenuous physical exercise. I now called this combination Endurance Caps because I have many marathon runners who use these capsules throughout their race.

Caution: Algae and seaweed are hydrophilic which means they attract water, algae and seaweeds absorbs liquid then expands to several times their size. Because of this ability it is important to drink lots of water when taking capsules that contain spirulina and kelp for instance. I found this out the hard way when being a lazy person I put my one teaspoon of nettle/kelp combo powder in a small glass of water rather than make a blended smoothie in which I used a cup of juice and yogurt. I tried to down the water/nettle/kelp combo but it stuck to my throat. I remember this well because as I was choking over the kitchen sink trying to get the clumped powder that was sticking to the sides of my throat, my teenage daughter walked by and said in a disgusted tone "Mom, you are so weird". I felt rather stupid actually. Make sure you use enough liquid when taking seaweed supplements.

Natural Salt

When I first tried to convince people to spend six bucks on a package of Celtic Salt, they thought me mad. Why spend money on salt when it cost next to nothing in the grocery store and besides salt wasn't good for you anyway. Today there are stores devoted to the different kinds of natural salt. Using a natural salt for your health bears repeating though.

Using salt that has been harvested from the sea and not stripped of its minerals such as Celtic salt from France which is harvested from salt flats near the sea by hand is better than ordinary table salt. If you look at the label of a package of Celtic salt you see a variety of minerals and micro minerals contained in the salt. The body needs all sorts of minerals for optimal health and in many cases in very small amounts so using a natural salt is a good way to obtain them.

My husband said that after he worked out at the gym he would sweat faster and more profusely if he was using Celtic salt rather than regular table salt. Table salt is sodium chloride, it has been stripped of all the minerals before packaging. Nowadays natural salt is easy to find.

Although I used Celtic salt for years I am now using Himalayan Pink Salt. Check out the different salt varieties and start using natural salt in your diet.

Fermented Foods

Every culture has some type of fermented food that is consumed on a regular basis not just for flavor but for its health benefits. Yogurt is an example of a fermented food which has become extremely popular in the US. The Germans swear by their sauerkraut which is fermented cabbage. I knew a young man suffering from Crohn's disease that swore by its digestives benefits as well. Kimchi is a fermented vegetable mixture from the Korean culture. I see that all types of fermented vegetables are now being sold at my famer's market. These cultured vegetables are also called lacto- fermented vegetables.

They are several methods to make fermented foods. Basically you soak raw vegetables in salted water and they ferment, creating a delicious tasting vegetables but more importantly the fermentation process creates certain bacteria that help promote the balance of healthy bacteria in the digestive system. The bacteria are called probiotic bacteria as opposed to antibiotic bacteria: pro life as opposed to anti life. Our digestive system contains all kinds of "good" and "bad" bacteria and we want to make sure that it has the right kind of bacteria for optimal digestion. Fermented foods with their "good" bacteria are a ticket to good digestion. If you have been taking antibiotic drugs it is smart to use these foods to reestablish the "good" bacteria during and after your illness.

My grandmother used vinegar and salt to make her pickles but this is different than the fermenting process. The salt creates a brine which makes nutrients, enzymes and probiotic bacteria from the raw foods. Incorporating a small amount of "fermented " foods in your daily diet helps the digestive process which in turn creates good health.

Sandor Elix Katz has written two great books on fermentation. His book "Wild Fermenting, The Flavors, Nutrition, and Craft of Live-Culture Foods" contains instructions and recipes along with his adventures in learning how to ferment just about any food and beverage. His latest " The Art of Fermentation, An In-depth Exploration of Essential Concepts and Processes from around the World" contains just about anything you would want to know about making fermenting foods and beverages. Both books are well worth reading.

Although they are not necessary there are several fermenting kits on the market that help the home cook make fermented foods if the process sounds too daunting. I use a kit that uses an airlock devise in the lid which in turns screws into a quart size canning jar. It makes fermenting small quantities of vegetables very easy. I found that I make foolproof fermenting recipes in a quantity that works for my needs. I have tried in the past to make sauerkraut and have failed dismally with an ordinary crock. I was more than discouraged after spending all that time shredding my garden grown cabbage. There are special pickling crocks available for larger quantities of vegetables with seals in their covers that ensure that the fermentation process works properly. There are very concise directions as well as videos detailing the fermentation process out there in books and on the internet these days.

My friend has access to whey, a by product of making cheese and yogurt, (she milks a cow) which she says makes wonderful fermented foods. The" Nourishing Traditions" cookbook has information and recipes on fermented foods using whey as a fermented medium instead of salt brine.

Kombucha Beverage

When I was learning about the herbs in the backwoods of Vermont, Massachusetts and New York there was this mysterious drink from Russia that was supposed to cure all ills. It was shrouded in mystery, you had to use white sugar (god forbid) and ordinary tea (god forbid) to make it and it grew mushrooms which you had to keep giving away. It felt like too much of a responsibility. Kombucha is a drink derived from a fungus which has been used throughout Europe and Asia for centuries and has been extensively studied because of its health benefits. Now this popular beverage Kombucha being sold in my local supermarket in all kinds of flavors and obviously it is very helpful . Who would have thought it would go mainstream? If you look at the label on Kombucha beverage you will see that it contains mega doses of probiotic bacteria similar to the probiotic bacteria that is contained in yogurt. Probiotic bacteria is extremely helpful in balancing the digestive system. So that might explain some of its immense popularity because digestive issues are people's biggest health complaint.

Fungi

Chaga is a charred looking growth that appears on birch trees here in the north woods. It has been harvested in other northern countries for centuries for its health and curing abilities. The use of Chaga tea has become very popular as of late. I see Chaga soap and cream as well as beverages being sold.

I have witnessed Reishi mushroom tincture as being helpful for allergies sufferers The health benefits of mushrooms is just starting to be understood and researched in this country. Ancient cultures revered certain species as longevity tonics. The Fungi family or mushrooms have been used throughout history for food and medicine. Officially fungi are not classified as plants but are in a category of their own, as this family should be. Paul Stamets who lives in Washington State has written and lectured extensively about this fascinating world. His company's Fungi Perfecti catalog and his website (www.fungi.com) are an encyclopedia of knowledge on all things fungi. I highly recommend browsing through his articles, videos and recipes, regardless of whether you are interested in using mushrooms. Their contribution to our planet's eco system is an eye opener.

An aside: The old adage "There are Old mushroom pickers and there are Bold mushrooms pickers but there are no Old, Bold mushroom pickers" still stands. Do not pick and eat mushrooms in the wild unless you have been out with an mushroom expert and you are positively sure about the identification. Many species of mushrooms are poisonous and people die after eating them.

Check out how to grow mushrooms with a mushrooms kit. There are available in many garden catalogs.

Chapter 18
GOOD FOOD CHOICES

Carbohydrate & Fiber-rich Foods

Grains with gluten: Wheat, Rye, Oats, Barley
Grains without gluten: Corn, Rice, Millet, Quinoa, Amaranth
Oatmeal - Regular or Steel cut
Potatoes, Sweet Potatoes
Rice, Brown Rice, Wild Rice
Legumes: All Beans (Kidney, Black, Pinto), Peas, Lentils, Chickpeas
Beets, Parsnips, Squashes

Protein-rich Foods

Beef, Beefalo, Buffalo, Lamb, Pork
Poultry: Chicken, Cornish Game Hens, Duck, Turkey
Fish, Cold Water fish: Salmon, Mackerel
Nuts and Seeds: Sesame, Almonds, Walnuts, Sunflower Seeds and Nut Butters
Peanuts and Peanut Butter
Eggs
Dairy: Yogurt, Milk, Cheese
Soy Foods: Tofu, Tempeh, Miso

Grains, Brown Rice, Beans, Corn, Barley, Amaranth, Quinoa
Algaes: Spirulina, Kelp
Barley, Wheat Grass and other Green vegetable Powders
Mushrooms
Broths made from bones

Vitamin, Mineral, Fiber- rich Foods

Vegetables raw and cooked
Leafy Green Vegetables: Lettuces, Swiss chard, Chicory
Cabbage, Broccoli, Cauliflower
Root Vegetables: Carrots, Beets, Turnips, Potatoes, Sweet Potatoes
Squashes: Butternut, Acorn, Pumpkin
Tomatoes, Peppers (Green, Red), Eggplant
Onions, Garlic, Leeks
Sea Vegetables: Nori, Hiziki, Kelp
Think of a rainbow selection when eating vegetables–vary the colors and the type of vegetables, below and above ground vegetables

Mushrooms

All types of mushrooms, Portabello, Shitake, etc.

Fruit

All kinds of Fruit particularly Fruit in Season
Dried Fruit
Frozen Fruit: Blueberries, Raspberries

Fats and Oil

Olive Oil cold pressed virgin oil stored in dark container
Sesame Oil
Coconut Oil
Safflower Oil
Grape seed Oil

Almond Oil
Walnut Oil
Flax Seed Oil (refrigerated)
Butter
Ghee
Nuts and Seeds
Meats
Cold water Fish: Salmon, mackerel, sardines

Salt

Sea salt
Himalayan Salt
Natural salts

Sweeteners

Honey
Molasses
Raw Sugar
Stevia

Fermented Foods - (lacto-fermented)

Yogurt
Kombucha Beverage
Sauerkraut
Fermented vegetables
Kimchi
Miso

Beverages

Water
Tea
Green Tea

Herbal Tea
Coffee
Milk
Coconut Milk
Almond Milk
Fruit juices
Water with lemon or lime slices
Seltzer water with ginger syrup or other syrups
Seltzer water with fruit juices
Herbal Teas with fruit juices

Condiments

Tamari
Soy Sauce
Culinary Herbs
Peppers
Garlic
Onions
Chili and Hot Sauces

Chapter 19

HERBS AS DIETARY SUPPLEMENTS

In the past, herbal plants were classified as food and regulated by the United States Department of Agriculture: they fell into the food category called GRAS, or "generally regarded as safe". They were reclassified in 1979, and are now regulated by the Federal Drug Agency. Today, herbal plants and botanical medicines are classified as "dietary supplements" alongside vitamins, minerals, and other combinations of substances touted as natural. I do not believe that plants should be classified as dietary supplements. They are not like chemical vitamins or the many other varieties of substances that make up this billion dollar industry. But then again, the marijuana plant is classified as a schedule 1 drug (another schedule 1 drug: heroin), so I can't say that I'm surprised.

I am often asked about what to take and how much to take of vitamins, minerals, and different supplements, but just because I have studied the science of nutrition does not mean I am trained in the use of vitamins as a healing therapy. I use plants for nutrition and medicine. My area of expertise is plants and plant preparations.

As I have stated before, Mark Pedersen chemically analyzes the nutritional profile of hundreds of herbs and foods in his book, *Nutritional Herbology*. It is full of charts and will satisfy your need to know.

Recommended Dietary Allowances

The Food and Nutrition Board (FNB) of the National Academy of Sciences prepares charts that reflect the amounts of vitamins, minerals and calories a person needs in order to avoid vitamin deficiencies. It is called the Recommended Dietary Allowances or RDA. If you look on the back of your vitamin pill bottle you will see the percentage of RDA or Daily Value that the vitamin contains along with the dosage of the pill or capsule. For instance, on a bottle of magnesium I see that one pill contains 400 mg and that that is considered to be 100% of my Daily Value. Every supplement label contains this type of information.

When I took nutrition courses in the 90s there was a big controversy about the dosage level for vitamins insofar as RDA charts offered information about vitamin *deficiencies*, not proper intake levels. Taking extremely large daily doses of vitamins and minerals had become very popular at the time. In response to this trend, the Food and Nutrition Board was in the process of developing the Recommended Daily Intake (RDI) chart, another set of guidelines that would suggest the proper amounts of vitamins and minerals to ingest in order to maintain optimal health. In 2017, this chart is called Adequate Intake, or AI. Tolerable Upper Intake Level, or UL, has been developed to suggest the maximum daily dosage that should be taken.

As with most nutritional vitamin information, no one can agree on the current dosage standards of vitamins for optimal health, but it essential to stay informed about the latest studies particularly since too high a dose can be harmful to the health. I am continually amazed by how high a dosage of vitamins people will take daily. They might be taking a multivitamin pill alongside other supplements that also contain the same vitamins, so they end up taking a very large daily dosage of certain vitamins. The body removes certain water soluble vitamins through the waste processes but not the fat soluble vitamins.

In this country, vitamins are added by law to bread, cereal and milk products. Bread and grain products receive added B vitamins and Folic acid; Milk products receive added vitamin A and D. If you have eliminated certain food groups from your diet such as grains, keep in mind that you must be conscious of adding those missing nutrients from other sources. For example, non-gluten diets are very popular at the moment, so the lack of grains also means a lack of vitamin B complex and fiber, both which are very important for the body. In the past, non-fat diets were popular but fat is an important nutrient for the body and people had skin problems as well as other conditions because of the lack of fats in their diets.

Best Ever Dietary Supplement

In the 80s, a blue green algae product called "Super Blue Green Am Algae" (*Aphanizaomenon flos-aquae*) was touted as the most nutritional food on earth. The company Cell Tech was a multimillion dollar company which sold dietary supplements through a multilevel marketing strategy, best known as pyramid scheme. It seemed that everyone and their mother was trying to sell you a bottle of these capsules. *Aphanizaomenon flos-aquae* is a genus of the cyanobacteria group of the Algae plant family. This particular strain was being grown on Lake Klamath in Oregon. Over time emerged a question about the safety of this product because this particular strain of cyanobacteria can produce a toxic byproduct if the water quality in which it is grown is not pure.

I remember this controversy very well because I compared the nutritional claims of this particular strain of blue green algae or cyanobacteria to claims about spirulina and nettles in a paper for my college botany class. At the time, many magazine articles (this was pre-internet) questioned the safety of Super Blue Green Am Algae. Because so many people had invested their money in this company and its products, its integrity and positive image became a very big deal to the people who wanted to continue to sell their inventory. At the time, it seemed that all the reports about product safety and the testing results were produced by the company itself, not by independent sources, so it was hard to figure out what was going on. The company is no longer in operation.

This "miracle" algae is not the only best-ever dietary supplement, of course. Several years ago, a type of calcium made from sea coral exploded on the market. It was touted as the only type of calcium to take and would cure all types of conditions. There was tremendous marketing for this particular type of calcium. The trouble was that it was not good for many people who were allergic to shellfish: people developed allergic symptoms when taking the coral calcium. Although this calcium might work for many people, it is not the only type of calcium supplement on the market.

Essential oils are the latest dietary supplement product being marketing very aggressively by means of a multi-level approach. Essential oil is the plant preparation used in Aromatherapy. I see similar patterns in the aggressive marketing of these products as used by the people who sold the Cell Tech blue green algae product. I am often bombarded by people who want to sell me bottles of this or that particular company's brand of essential oils. According to the "experts", *their* company is the only company on Earth that makes a therapeutic essential oil that works—no other essential oil companies are any good. I have also noticed that classes are being taught on the medicinal use of these particular essential oil blends. It is important to ask about the teacher's experience with and training regarding the products that they are teaching about. Does their aromatherapy education derive only from the company? Have they studied Aromatherapy? (Aromatherapy is a certified course in this country.) People buy the kits and of course want to make returns on their investment. Are they teaching the course in order to sell those particular products?

These are just three examples of the" latest and greatest" super foods or dietary supplements I have seen, three items that are going to provide you with everything you need to be healthy in a convenient, capsule-like preparation. The issues of safety, properly labeled contents, and marketing must be addressed. It seems like wherever we look these days, someone touts him or herself as an expert in all things wellness.

What's in the bottles?

Every couple of years a news report surfaces geared to frighten consumers about the dangers of using botanical supplements. The latest scare report was issued by the New York Attorney General. In this report, the department stated that the contents of certain herbal supplement bottles did not match what was stated on the label. They used a new type of testing using DNA to verify that the contents of the bottles of certain plants.

Looking further into this study (as did The Natural Product Association), I found that there was no other information about how they conducted their research or about this new testing method. Which herbs were tested? What was stated on the labels? Where did they purchase the bottles of herbs? As of the writing of this book, they still haven't released the details of the report.

As a result of this "study", people could only hear that there were ground-up houseplants instead of the herbs stated on the label in the supplement bottles issued by GMC and Walmart. As there is supposedly no regulation at all in this industry, they heard that they should not trust any herbal companies or herb supplements.

Chromatography

There are many different types of chromatography testing for plants. We hear a lot about the testing of plants because testing is used extensively these days to test the ratio of THC and CBD levels in medical marijuana. So I wondered what type of DNA testing was used in the study mentioned above and if it was the best testing method for plants. Additionally, there is extensive regulation in the dietary supplement industry but, as usual, it is up to the consumer to be aware. We have an incredible research engine at our fingertips so there is no excuse not to become informed about what you are using.

The website of the American Herbal Products Association (ahpa.org) issued this response to the New York Attorney General office's survey on herbal dietary supplements:

"All facilities that manufacture herbal supplements are required by U.S. law to comply with strict current good manufacturing practice (cGMP) requirements that are enforced by the FDA. These cGMP requirements mandate that manufacturers have proper controls in place to ensure the quality of their dietary supplement products and to help assure consumers that they get accurately labeled and unadulterated dietary supplements. One section of the cGMP requirements directs manufacturers to verify the identity of dietary ingredients, including botanical ingredients, and document the testing used to verify identity. FDA regularly inspects dietary supplement manufacturing facilities to ensure compliance with cGMP requirements and has authority to take action to protect consumers when products are not manufactured in compliance with cGMP requirements and could pose a danger to consumers."

Safety of herbal supplements

Questioning the safety of the products that are being sold in the supplement industry is a huge concern to everyone these days, as it should be. It is important to research the companies and their products.

The internet has made things easier in this regard but also more confusing given the plethora of information you'll find. It is like the food that you ingest: know your source.

I grow my own plants, make my own medicines or get my herbs and herbal products from reputable companies who abide by strict regulations for their manufacturing procedures and products.

Look it up: Internet Search Engines and your Local Library

Most people get all their information from internet search engines. When checking out supplement information, check out the origin of the web site that you are reading. If the website from which you are obtaining the information is the company's website, explore other opinions. Check out independent websites that that are not invested in selling the products that you are interested in. The Natural Products Association and the American Herbal Product Association are very involved in making sure that this industry is safe and thriving. The Natural Products Association website (www.npainfo.org) has information on all kinds of supplements and their manufacturers, as well as other important information that pertains to this huge industry. The American Botanical Council is an organization that has been researching and staying on top of all the latest information about herbal products. They publish an excellent publication called Herbalgram. Their website is www.herbalgram.org which contains a wealth of information about the herbal world.

There are three government agencies whose websites have extensive information on Dietary Supplements: the National Institute of Health: www.nih.gov; the United States Department of Agriculture: www.usda.gov; and the Federal Drug Agency: www.fda.gov. These sites offer the latest information about nutrition and the safety of the food and supplements that are on the market along with an incredible amount of information about health.

The FDA website also has a special page through which you can check out any pharmaceutical, drug, herb, or other supplement: www.nlm.nih.govv/medlineplus/druginformation. This is also where you can report any adverse effects of dietary supplements. I recommend taking the time to report problems because this is how they compile the information on particular supplements; it is just as important as reporting any adverse pharmaceutical drug reactions because the same holds true with drugs.

A place that is often overlooked in this era of electronic devises is the local library and the knowledgeable librarians who are versed in researching information. I give my local library my herbal book lists and they are grateful to know what herbal books to order.

cGMP

In 2007, the FDA established new manufacturing guidelines for the dietary supplement industry: although the GMP (Good Manufacturing Processes) had been in place before, the standards were revised to incorporate the new available technologies. cGMP stands for current Good Manufacturing Process, which is the new standard for manufacturing facilities. The Natural Products Association website (www.npainfo.org) has information about specific manufacturers and their compliance with the new regulations.

Latin Names to Identify the Herbal Plants

All bottles of herbal plants must use the Latin name of the plant. Latin is the universal language of plant identification. I had never felt as helpless as I did one afternoon in my local health food store when I tried to figure out which digestive herb a Russian gentleman needed: he didn't speak much English and only knew the common Russian name of the herb. I knew about the herbs that helped digestion but I didn't know the Russian names. The Latin name, or universal name, would have solved all our translation problems (and his stomach ache).

Recently, I have encountered bottles of herbal supplements that have been sold to patients by their doctors without proper labels. The label on the bottle should have the Latin name of the herb, not just the common name of the herb. One of the bottles I have come across only uses the common names of the herbs—and they are in German. This sort of thing makes it difficult to research the herbal formula.

Labeling

The FDA has strict labeling requirements for dietary supplements. They are currently being revised. The label should include name of the product, who made/packed/distributed it, the serving size, all of the ingredients and their amounts (including fillers, binders and flavors), the expiration date, the nutritional content of the ingredients, and the percentage of the DV (Daily Value) of those ingredients.

As we have seen in the past, the label cannot contain any claims that the product can cure, mitigate, treat or prevent disease. Accordingly to the FDA, only drugs can use those claims. Again, this can be a difficult grey area if you are using supplements to enhance your health. We won't go down the GMO labeling fight that is currently ongoing in this country since a huge percentage of the population would like to see GMO (Genetically Modified Organism) food labeled as such.

Marketing Techniques of Dietary Supplements

Cell Tech used a pyramid type of marketing to sell its popular products. Many popular dietary supplement companies continue to use this type of marketing, but the drawbacks of multi-level marketing, sometimes called pyramid schemes, are clear. When a person invests their money into a product that they must sell personally, they lose their objectivity. They are interested in selling their product and although they might believe in the product, the bottom line is that they want to sell the product.

I have seen this scenario repeat itself over and over throughout my years as an herbalist. I used to receive so many cassette tapes and literature in the mail, as well as personal sales pitches that touted the latest natural product that was going to change the world.

I use plants which grow in my backyard: why I am the target of all this advertising remains a mystery to me.

Health Professionals Selling Dietary Supplements

For many years, chiropractors have been in the business of selling high cost supplements to their patients. I have noticed lately that physicians have started to sell all kinds of supplements out of their offices at very high markups as well. This is a slippery slope for patients and their healthcare providers. In the recent past, doctors were not allowed to sell medicines out of their offices: that was the job of the pharmacist and the drug store. There is a reason for separating the two activities: it's a conflict of interest. Like the person involved in multi-level marketing, the doctor cannot objectively market or prescribe the product because they are personally invested in selling it—regardless of how much they believe in the product.

In addition, the dietary supplements sold by physicians are very expensive: over the course of time, these become unaffordable to many of their patients. Please note that most of the products that are being sold out of these offices are available at a much lesser cost from stores and by mail order.

Body Building Industry

One of the biggest misuses of dietary supplements is that of the use of supplements for the purpose of body building. Young men consume all types of supplements and powders to bulk up their muscle mass and increase their energy so that they can have a stronger "work out". They use protein powders to increase their calorie intake without eating food. The ingredient lists of these powders are extensive. In my nutrition class, I remember how interested some of my students were in what they could take to build up their bodies. In one class, these young Marines were very curious, but they were also very aware of the dangers caused by some of the chemicals found in their daily supplements regimen. They were just interested in how long they could take certain substances before they would affect the liver. They knew about cycling on and off these substances every six weeks. I was amazed by their knowledge about the supplement world. But most young people do not know that these supplement powders affect their livers and every part of their anatomy. Many of these powders contain testosterone-type substances and affect their emotional and mental attitudes as well.

Weight Loss Industry

The other misuse of dietary supplements is that of the use of such supplements for weight loss. The money involved in the manufacture of weight loss products and procedures is staggering. The herbal world is not exempt from promoting the latest and greatest weight loss plant. When people used to ask me, I would tell them that if there were any herbs for losing weight—if I had figured out an herbal blend that could create weight loss—I would be a very wealthy woman living in a beach house in Hawaii.

In the mid-nineties, Herbalife, a multi-level marketing billion dollar company, sold a weight loss product that was extremely popular. It came with two bottles, green and beige, and you used the green pills during the day and the beige pills at night. The green bottle contained several herbs that worked as stimulants. The first listed herb, Ma Huang, is the plant Ephedra: this herb works to curb the appetite and boost the energy in the body.

The Ephedra plant comes from the Chinese tradition and is used for respiratory conditions. It helps open up the lungs so that people can breathe better. It also boosts the metabolism of the body but has an adverse effect on the circulatory system, namely the heart, if used improperly or as a daily supplement. Ephedra does not work as a tonic herb; it is used for specific respiratory conditions. In this sense, it is a very useful herb to use if you are having an asthma attack. However, Ephedra was not being used in this way: instead, it was put into weight loss and body building products to create energy in the body without eating food. It raised the metabolism of the body while controlling or suppressing the appetite. Using stimulant herbs to create energy is what we do in this country with our love of coffee and Red Bull-type drinks.

The green bottle also contained Guarana, an herb that contains large amounts of caffeine as well as several urinary specific herbs that work as diuretics. The green pills gave a boost of energy while the diuretic herbs helped shed the water weight. The beige bottle contained the herb Valerian which is a strong sedative herb which works as a muscle relaxer and is a specific for heart palpitations. The beige pills also contained several herbs that worked as laxatives in the digestive system. I remember the calls I would get from women who were experiencing heart palpitations and other physical symptoms when using these diet pills. They were perplexed by their symptoms and wanted to know what was causing the problems. In short, yes, you did lose weight by taking these pills because you didn't eat real food and you dropped your water weight along with everything else. But at what cost to the body?

The sale of the herb Ephedra was banned in New York State in 2004 because of the problems associated with the side effects caused when used as a dietary supplement. Supplements that contain the active ingredients of Ephedra, ephedrine, are still available to purchase, but the sale of the plant itself has been banned.

Several years ago, my herb shop and the tea shop in the building where I work was inundated with women seeking four herbs. Pu-erh, White tea, Chickweed and Bilberry had been recommended by Dr. Oz for weight loss. These herbs come from different cultures and have been traditionally used for weight loss. On his talk show, Dr. Oz recommended that dieters drink several cups of all of these herbs every day to promote weight loss. The majority of the women seeking these herbs were elderly and probably taking pharmaceuticals drugs. The amount of tea that was supposed to be drunk (and the fact that several of the teas worked as diuretics) made me wonder how effective the strategy could be for their weight loss and metabolism. It is important to research the herbs that are suggested by these "experts" and then see if they work for you. Start with a low dosage: one or two cups a day. It is hard to determine what works if you just start by taking four different herbs several times a day. I see the desperation that people feel about weight gain all the time. But these quick fixes rarely work.

Exploitation of Lyme patients

The latest disease or condition that is being exploited by many healthcare professionals is Lyme disease. It is a very confusing condition to all—the people who have it and the people who treat it. The exploitation of these very vulnerable people is heartbreaking. To me it represents all that is broken within our healthcare system. The medical community cannot agree on the proper treatment, the tests are not consistent, the testing companies are compromised by conflicts of interest and the insurance companies are completely involved in deciding which drug treatments can be used based solely on cost. Different types of therapies are not covered under insurance plans so the affected person is extremely limited in seeking out other healing modalities. Then there are doctors who charge extraordinary out of pocket fees to see Lyme patients. They recommend a smorgasbord of drugs and dietary supplements and sell the supplements themselves at a premium.

Testimonials

Testimonials are just that: People quoted as saying that the supplement really worked for them or that it was the answer to every health problem they ever had. Advertisements are filled with testimonials. Just understand that what works for some people might not be the right strategy (or supplement) for you. Do not let anyone tell you that there is something amiss with you because that particular supplement or, for that matter, drug, did not help you. It doesn't work that way. We are all individuals and have individual needs.

Training in the Use of Dietary Supplements and Botanical Medicine

Don't be shy, ask about the training and experience that your doctor, chiropractor, nutritionist, acupuncturist, aromatherapist, massage therapist, psychotherapist or herbalist has received in regard to the products they are suggesting. In my experience, physicians and chiropractors use a hit or miss approach to prescribing herbal and other dietary supplements because they have little training in the use of herbs, nutrition or vitamin therapy.

SECTION 3 | *Be Well, Stay Well*

In fact, most health practitioners (and this includes most alternative health practitioners as well) do not have training in nutrition or the medicinal use of plants.

Some of the worst herbal advice I have heard has come from the lips of "alternative health practitioners". Just because someone works in a different, non-mainstream modality of the medical world does not mean that they have any training in botanical medicine. In New York State, anyone can call themselves a nutritionist, but there are also board certified nutritionists in New York State: in other words, if you seek a nutritionist's expertise, ask about your nutritionist's credentials. Experience is very important, and I do not mean to suggest that only officially certified health practitioners are experts on health. Far from it. Currently in the United States we do not have a certified program for Botanical Medicine but people are using plants for food and medicine. I have spent my life learning my craft as have many, many others. Ask about your practitioner's education, training and experience.

Kinesiology as a Diagnostic Tool

I am trained in several techniques of energy work, or kinesiology. Reiki is a form of energy work that most people are familiar with. I am a huge proponent of energies techniques. They work. They help people in numerous ways and can be used as a diagnostic method.

There is a nutritionist's office in my town that uses a form of kinesiology to diagnose what type of supplements people need for their health. They test people by using an arm pushing technique. It has been my experience that although this testing method might say that a particular bottle of supplements could be good for their condition, this doesn't mean that they should take it. People leave from their appointments with a bag of supplement bottles.

Over the course of subsequent visits, I do not believe that the nutritionist tends to test which supplements are no longer needed for a person's condition. They just prescribe additional supplements. The result of this is that people spend hundreds of dollars every month on supplements and end up with hundreds of bottles of partially-used supplements. They spend so much money on supplements that they feel they are wasting money if they don't use up the bottles. So they take even more capsules or pills. I have noticed that many of these bottles contain similar vitamins, minerals and herbs, just in a different ratios under a different name. I have spent numerous consultations helping my clients add up the different substances that they are taking on a regular basis. They usually come to see me because they have digestive issues.

Digestion Issues

Pills and capsules are hard on the digestive system. They contain substances like fillers, binders and hard-to-digest substances. By ingesting supplements, we hope to enhance our health rather than create an obstruction to the digestive system. I have had people cover my massage table with all the bottles of supplements that they take daily. Sometimes they need two bags to bring in all the bottles. I started rating people as one or two baggers. Combine all the binders, fillers and the gelatin of the capsules that you are ingesting and you have a quantity of foreign substances in your GI tract. Such a regimen of supplements might be ok for a couple of months, but (depending on the person) problems will appear thereafter. I suggest emptying the capsules and grinding the pills and putting them into a shake or smoothie so that it is easier on the digestive system.

What am I taking and why?

My biggest problem with dietary supplements is that people have no idea what or why they are taking the supplement. I have seen this time and time again. Is it a ground up plant in a capsule? Is it a pill—and if it is a pill what kind of substance is in the binding or filler? Is it a combination of herbs, vitamins, and minerals or other chemicals? Are you taking a mega dose of vitamins when you add up the percentages? Are the herbs working or is it the vitamins? What is in the supplement powder? Do you read the label and see if there are any allergens in the list of ingredients?

There are so many paths to healing. If the standard of care in our medical system (which only uses drugs and surgery as tools) worked, there would not be a thriving world of alternative healing methods in this country. There would not be a billion dollar supplement market. There would not be herbalists who are trained in botanical medicine, chiropractors, nor acupuncturists, never mind such a range of practitioners of all the energy healing modalities. It is time to recognize other healing therapies and include them in our medical system.

Innate Wisdom of our Bodies

We possess an innate understanding of what is good to eat and drink and what not to eat or drink for our particular body. We are individuals with individual needs. You might say, "I know I shouldn't be eating this but I can't help myself," but yes, you can. It's a choice. I have seen people take charge of their health and listen to their body's needs and return to a state of health and wellbeing. There is so much conflicting information about diets, healthy foods, and cooking methods that it is easy to get overwhelmed. Start with the food you eat on a daily basis. I have learned that it is the foods and drinks that you eliminate from your diet that make all the difference in one's health. I always say, "Spend your money on good food and you won't spend it on medicines." That includes dietary supplements.

As a child, I had an exotic aunt that lived in New York City. She came to our house for the holidays. She was on a very strange diet called the macrobiotic diet that had some pretty weird food in it. She introduced our family to "brown rice," which was so strange to us kids who had only ever encountered white rice and that was only on the rare occasion when we "ate out" at a Chinese restaurant. We were from Maine and ate potatoes at just about every meal. She knew George Oshawa, the founder of the macrobiotic diet, personally. She touted the diet to be the cure of all health problems, the greatest diet ever. She felt great and looked great. But at no time did this stop her from heartily enjoying the turkey dinners served at Thanksgiving or the ham at Easter. She was a French Canadian woman through and through, and loved and enjoyed eating with gusto. That's what you want to aspire to: Eat, Drink and be Merry.

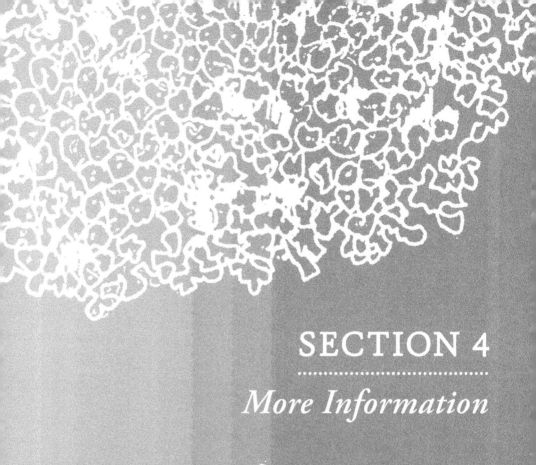

SECTION 4

More Information

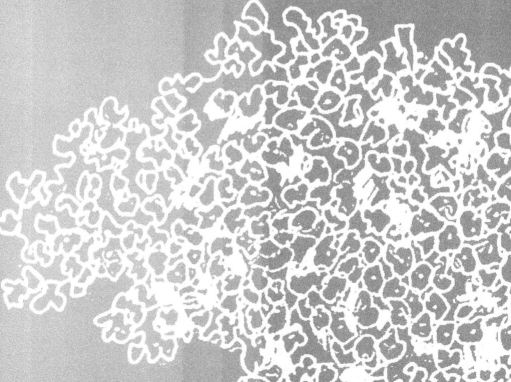

Chapter 20

ABOUT THE PLANTS
MATERIA MEDICA

In every serious herbal book (or "Herbal", as they can be called) is a section called "Materia Medica", meaning material one uses for medicine. In an herbal book, the "material" is obviously that of the plants themselves.

It is important to understand the individual plants and how they affect the body. By looking up each plant individually, one can develop a broader understanding of a plant's actions and the functions of associated herbal recipes. Please acquaint yourself with "Materia Medica" written by several different herbalists.

I have divided up the information in my "Materia Medica" into:

- *Name:* Common Name and Latin Name

- *Part Used:* The part of the plant you use: root, flower, or leaf.

- *Collection:* When to collect and harvest the plant.

- *Found:* Is the plant found in the wild or is it cultivated in a garden

- *Growing:* The optimal environment in which to grow the plant: does the plant prefer a dry soil or a moist soil? (Based on my humble experience: it is not the *only* experience.)

- *Actions:* How the plant affects the body. Refer to the **Language of Plants** section.

- *Body:* What part of the body the plant affects.

- *Use:* The history of use.

☞ *Experience:* My personal experience with using the plant.

☞ *Preparation:* The best way to use the plant: tea, tincture, syrup etc.

When my ethnobotanist officemate decides what herbs he needs for a health issue, he looks up the plant and its chemical constituents in the "Materia Medica" of an herbal book that contains that scientific information. He first studies the chemical constituent that has been scientifically-proven to work for that particular health condition. For example, when he needs an anti-inflammatory herb he knows that the constituent curcumin is recognized by the scientific community for its anti-inflammatory properties. Turmeric becomes his choice because of the large amount of curcumin that is contained in the root.

Studying the "Material Medica" section in herbals, particularly those found in older books, is very helpful when attempting to understand plants and how they can help.

Boneset *Eupatorium perfoliatum*

Part Used: Leaves and Flowers

Collection: Pick in late summer just before the flowers open

Found: Wild: edges of wetlands, riverbanks, fields (very common in our area)

Growing: Perennial. Transplants well in a garden setting depending on the soil's ability to retain water. Although I grow it in my sandy soil in my home garden, it also grows in the clay soil in my big medicinal garden. It is truly a wetlands plant and flourishes along the riverbanks all over my area.

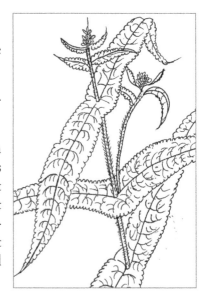

Actions: Anti-microbial, Diaphoretic, Anti-spasmodic

Body: Respiratory, Immune

Use: Long history of relieving the symptoms of the flu particularly for "breakbone fever" where your bones ache. Helps with the aches and pains associated with the flu and has a strong anti-viral action. Key ingredient in flu remedies.

Experience: I think it is the best plant for reducing the symptoms of the flu. I combine it with Elder Flower, Yarrow, Peppermint, and Catnip to make a good-tasting infusion that really helps with flu. It has a bitter taste so it is best to combine it with other plants. I have found that the taste is not a problem when people are sick as they can't taste it anyway; it works so very well in alleviating that miserable feeling of being sick.

Preparation: Infusion, Tincture, Bath

Calendula *Calendula officinalis*

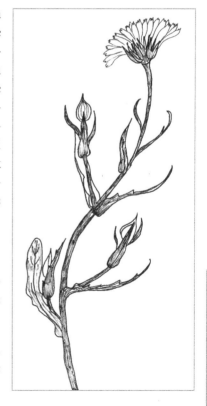

Marigold is the English (U.K.) common name for Calendula. In the U.S., the name marigold refers to a completely different species (Tagetes) which is a very popular garden flower. Because so many herbal books are from the United Kingdom, it is easy to confuse the two flowers and think that our common garden flower is really the medicinal species of Calendula. Make sure you check the plant tag for the Latin name of Calendula officinalis when purchasing seeds or plants to be sure of the correct plant.

Part Used: Flowers

Collection: Pick flowers, let mature flowers go to seed. Collect dried flowerheads for their seed (it self-sows)

Found: Cultivated: seeds found in garden centers and in catalogs. Ask a friend for the dried flowerheads which contain the seeds.

Growing: Very easy plant to grow. It flowers from early summer to late fall. Beautiful, cheerful plant. There are many cultivators out there now. Make sure you are growing the medicinal species. The flowers produce a resin which leaves hands sticky when picking.

Actions: Antimicrobial, Antiseptic, Anti-inflammatory

Body: Skin, Respiratory, Immune

Use: Because of its strong antimicrobial properties, it is a good addition to infusions for cold and flu remedies. It is a specific for skin imbalances.

Experience: I use the flowers in respiratory recipes because of its highly antiseptic properties. It is an important part of my Sinus Steam. It is one of the most effective plants for skin imbalances or "weird skin thingies". The homeopathic calendula cream on the market has helped many sufferers of skin rashes. I have found that the oil works well for all types of skin issues.

Preparation: Infusion, Bath, Compress, Oil

Catnip *Nepeta cataria*

Part Used: Leaves and Flowers

Collection: Pick anytime throughout growing season. Mint family rule: best picked when flowering.

Found: Wild: Fields, Gardens

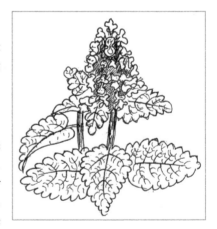

Growing: I transplant the catnip babies to my medicinal garden in the spring. Catnip pops up everywhere in early spring and later in the fall in our area. It can become a large plant so make sure you give it room to grow: it will shade out other plants. It can be transplanted in the fall for the next year. No one complains if you harvest this plant from their gardens as it is considered a weed. It can be cut several times during the growing season.

Actions: Diaphoretic, Sedative, Carminative

Body: Respiratory, Immune, Nervous, Digestive

Use: Catnip is a member of mint family. Like many mint plants, its smell is very complex. It helps the digestive system, calms the nervous system, and reduces fever (especially in children). It is very safe. I use it in my Traditional Gypsy Remedy. To cats it acts as a stimulant, but catnip has the opposite effect on humans.

Experience: I make sure to have fresh dried catnip on hand every year since I have five grandchildren. This is a very good plant for children and their imbalances. Children get sick without a lot of first signs or warnings (and get better very fast). A cup of catnip tea helps them calm down and move the illness out of their system quickly. I use catnip infusion in a hot bath which is an effective preparation for children as well as adults.

Preparation: Infusion, Tincture, Bath

Cayenne *Capsicum fructescens*

Part Used: Fruit

Collection: When pepper is ripe it turns red. In the Northeast, this occurs at end of summer and into fall.

Found: Cultivated

Growing: Peppers grow very well in the Northeast, but need sufficient water and summer heat. It is important to make sure they have enough sunlight in the garden. The plants should be started in-

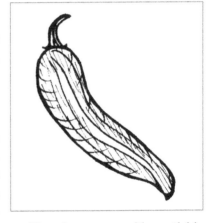

doors because they have a long growing time. The plants are readily available in garden centers because cayenne is popular for culinary use. Make sure you are buying the correct species when buying cayenne peppers. People are devoted to all kinds of hot peppers so gardens centers carry many different types. I have never had a problem with a mismarked species of cayenne because of its popularity. They can be grown in containers—in fact, they do very well in containers—just make sure the containers are big enough.

Actions: Stimulant, Carminative, Tonic, Antiseptic

Body: Whole Body, Circulatory, Immune, Skin, Digestive

Use: Used as a stimulant for the whole body. It is particularly useful when the cold or flu tends to linger in the system. Cayenne helps regulate blood flow throughout the body, strengthening the heart and the capillaries: in this way, it works as a tonic for the circulatory system. Externally, it helps relieve muscular and nerve pain.

Experience: I use powdered cayenne in my cold caps and yellow pills as a stimulant to help move illness out of the body. It is used as a tonic for the circulatory system. See the nervous system section for more information on herbal stimulants. It can be used as gargle for a sore throat, but that is only for the brave.

Preparation: Food, Infusion, Tincture, Gargle, Cream, Oil

Chamomile *Matricaria chamomilla*

Part Used: Flowers

Collection: Pick as flowers mature and form large seed heads, all season long.

Found: Gardens, wild. If you are picking it from the wild make sure you correctly identify it. In the Northeast, people mistake pineapple weed (*Matricaria discoidea*, a very common plant) and other lookalikes for wild chamomile.

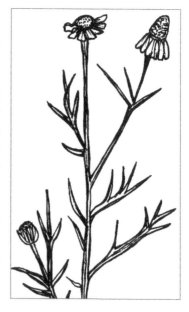

Growing: Once growing it will reseed in the garden, leading many to believe it to be a perennial. Easy to grow from seed. Transplant babies to wherever you want them in your garden. Caution: rabbits really like it.

Actions: Nervine, Anti-spasmodic, Carminative, Bitter, Anti-inflammatory, Antimicrobial

Body: Nervous, Digestive

Use: Works on two body systems (nervous and digestive). It is rich in essential oils which are activated by steaming or using it in an herbal bath. Studied extensively by the scientific community.

Experience: One of my favorite plants in my category of "strong but gentle" herbs. We have a misguided notion that plant actions have to be strong in order to be effective. Chamomile has persisted in the general consciousness for so long as a benign herbal tea (After all, Peter Rabbit drank it, so how powerful could it be?) A cup of chamomile tea can be a comfort when sick. Because it calms you down and helps to digest your food at the same time, it makes a wonderful after-dinner drink. These same properties are so helpful when sick. It is very calming to children. I recommend steeping it for only 10-15 minutes. If steeped long enough the tea has a bitter flavor. Since bitterness is a specific for the digestive system, the bitter taste is perfectly good but not desirable for many people. I have found that people are amazed at how delicious fresh chamomile tastes. Their experience of chamomile usually derives from purchasing tea bags from the store. There is a big difference in flavor.

Preparation: Infusion (steep 10-15 minutes to avoid bitter flavor or for 1 hour to achieve its bitter principles), Tincture, Bath, Foot Bath, Poultice, Cream

Comfrey *Symphytum officinale*

Part Used: Leaves and Roots

Collection: Throughout growing season.

Found: Garden

Growing: Once established in the garden, comfrey is very prolific; it will spread by seeds as well. I watched as many comfrey plants popped up everywhere in the botanical garden that had been seeded by my com-

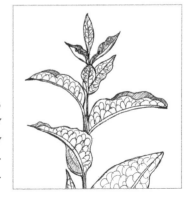

frey plants (much to other gardeners' dismay). This plant gets very large so plan on placing it in a corner of the garden. Once you put it anywhere it will continue to grow from the small pieces of roots it leaves behind.

Actions: Vulnerary, Demulcent, Astringent

Body: All mucous membranes, Respiratory, Skin

Use: History of external use for skin problems and healing of wounds. Contains allantoin which stimulates skin cell growth. Important to be careful when applying it to deep cuts as it closes wounds from the skin down which may create infections. It is not antimicrobial like calendula so it is combined with other anti-microbial herbs in a poultice. Although it has been used for thousands of years internally, it is important that you understand the controversy that surrounds it (see respiratory section on the comfrey controversy). It is also used for animal food.

Experience: I substitute marshmallow root for old herbal recipes—usually respiratory recipes—that call for the use of comfrey. I use comfrey leaves and roots externally. The roots are invaluable for so many skin issues. I make a Comfrey Fennel Eye Wash to help deal with eye infections. (See the **Preparation** section on eye washes.) The leaves make great poultices: ground up, they are filled with healing juices and are easy to apply.

Preparation: Powder (root and leaf), Poultices, Mask, Oils Infusion, Decoction (root), Salves

Echinacea: *Echinacea purpurea, Echinacea augustoflia, Echinacea pallida*

Part Used: Flowers, Leaves, Buds, Roots

Collection: Pick when plant is in full bloom; pick roots in fall.

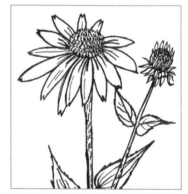

Found: Wild in prairies of the Midwest (U.S.A.); Cultivated in gardens in the Northeast.

Growing: The species *Echinacea purpurea* grows best in the Northeast. It grows very well in all types of soil. It can tolerate dry conditions but doesn't like wet soils. Sow from seed or by division. Beautiful addition to any garden.

The flower has become so popular that many differently colored and weirdly shaped flower cultivars are on the market. Make sure you buy the correct medicinal species, Echinacea purpurea. Check out the garden tags and look for the Latin name to correctly identify the species.

Actions: Preventative, Immunostimulant, Antimicrobial

Body: Immune, Skin, Respiratory

Use: A long history of use for colds, flu, and infections of the skin. Acts as a preventative, taken at the first signs of an imbalance; it will stimulate the body's defense mechanism and prevent the illness. Echinacea preparations are the most popular herbal medicine in Germany. It is recommended for use over the course of two weeks only (take a break after this period). It is very safe to use. It is important that you take it in a dose large enough to work: ½ - 1 tsp several times daily to prevent colds (depending on the person). Alcohol-based tincture is the preferred preparation.

Experience: I was taught in my early herbal schooling that tincturing the root of the augustofolia plant was the only way to use this versatile plant. I have since found that the stems, leaves, buds, and flowers of the purpurea species (the species that is used in Germany) make a very effective tincture. In fact, I rarely use the roots anymore. I was also taught that you should take only take the plant for two weeks, but my experience with Echinacea has been different.

When I teach, I conduct informal surveys about the ways in which people use Echinacea. Years ago, only a few people used Echinacea, but now most of the people in my classes use some type of Echinacea preparation. There are so many Echinacea products/preparations on the market now; when I ask which my students about which of these work, those who did not have good results identified that they had taken Echinacea pills, capsules or other preparations. In general, I recommend the alcohol or tincture preparation. When I ask, "How long do you take Echinacea?" most people report that they take their preparations for durations ranging from a couple days to two weeks at most.

Other people use Echinacea as a preventative because they work with the public. They take a tiny dose throughout the winter or cold season. They feel that it is very helpful used in this way. Since the weather of the cold season can be sporadic, they take breaks in their pattern of usage accordingly.

Echinacea was a plant favored by the eclectic doctors of the 1900s: as such, there is much information about the plant in old and new herbal medical texts alike. *Echinacea: Nature's Immune Enhancer by* Steven Foster explores the history of this wonderful, native plant as well as its contemporary uses.

Preparation: Capsules, Decoction, Tinctures, Poultices

Elder *Sambucus nigra*

Part Used: Berries, Flowers

Collection: Flowers in spring, berries when ripe (late summer, early Fall)

Found: Wild: fields, edges of wood, wetlands; Cultivated

Growing: Easy to grow if it gets enough water.

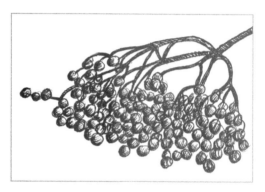

Caution: Birds love the ripe berries and can reach them before you can. There is nothing more discouraging than going out to pick ripe berries only to find that the birds got there first. Once, my friend and I went to pick berries when the bushes were filled with berries but when we checked bush after bush we saw that the birds had plucked all the ripe berries.

Elder bushes flourish in a neighboring county a little south of my region. It is also a farming area with many large cleared fields. The bushes are found along the woods line and scattered throughout open fields. Elder bushes do not fare as well here as we are further north, and just that much cooler and more forested. They grow ok for a couple of years, then die back. Check out the zone requirements in the gardening catalogs if you purchase elder bushes. Also make sure you are growing a medicinal species because there are several different species available. Once established they do well. I have beautiful elder bushes growing in my garden which has clay soil. I was surprised they fared so well but clay soil retains water so they are happy, much happier than they were in my sandy soil of my yard. Move the bushes around if you are having problems growing them. I have noticed they like to grow in front of the woods besides a cleared field.

Actions: Flowers: Diaphoretic, Anti-catarrhal. Berries: Tonic, Immunostimulant, Adaptagen, Diaphoretic

Body: Immune, Respiratory

Use: Ancient history of use of the whole plant: bark, leaves, flowers and berries. The flowers are used for respiratory imbalances; they combine well with yarrow, peppermint, catnip, and boneset to form an excellent formula for influenza. The berries make a great-tasting immunity syrup which is very popular (check out the recipe section). Both the berries and flowers help maintain the health of the immune system and work as preventatives of colds and the flu. The leaves are used for poultices.

Experience: I love this plant. I was so glad to find an herb that works as a preventative for winter imbalances that can be taken every day (and tastes good). The ripe berries of the elder bush fit this role. People love the taste of the berries which makes them compliant when it comes to taking their medicine. Children love the flavor of elderberries, especially when made into a syrup preparation. Mix different herbs or tinctures into the tea and syrup; the elderberry flavor disguises other tastes very well. The syrup is easy to make from dried berries. There is no need to buy it from the health food store. The flowers are harvested in spring: I use them in my Traditional Gypsy Flu Remedy.

Years ago I gave an herbal talk in a small rural library where the youngest person in the room was over 60. Everyone there was raised on elderberry pie and remembers as children how hard it was to remove the numerous berries from the stems which was their job. Fortunately the berries can be easily removed when you dry the berries on their stems. It is worth harvesting the berries and drying them: they keep well. A bush contains a lot of berries, I prefer to dry them and use them as needed. I make quarts of the syrup with the dried berries during the winter season. Of course, you can make elder syrup from fresh berries as well. In the recipe section I have listed several delicious recipes that use elderberries. This is a medicinal plant worth growing in your yard.

Preparation: Food, Infusion, Tincture, Syrup, Poultice

Elecampane *Inula helenium*

Part Used: Root

Collection: Dig root in fall

Found: Wild, Fields, Cultivated

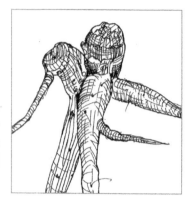

Growing: Grows very well in the garden. Tall, large plant with sunflower-like blossoms. Easy to transplant and easy to dig the roots in the fall. I have seen fields of wild elecampane growing in my area.

Action: Expectorant, Anti-tussive, Diaphoretic, Antiseptic, Anti-bacteria

Body: Respiratory, Digestive

Use: Long history of use for colds that cause respiratory imbalances. Elecampane helps soothe the cough reflex but also helps move the mucous of the lungs. It is a mild expectorant. It works well for children. The fresh root smells and tastes good. The taste gets stronger with age. It combines well with other herbal roots, as well as demulcent herbs like marshmallow root and/or licorice root.

Experience: Very helpful for coughs. It is not too strong and provides soothing and strong antimicrobial actions. I think this plant is extremely effective for respiratory imbalances. This is my favorite expectorant plant. I grow and harvest the root every season. Combined with marshmallow root, it makes a simple but effective cough recipe.

Preparation: Decoction, Cold Infusion, Tincture, Syrup

Fennel *Foeniculum vulgare*

Part Used: Leaves, Bulb, Seeds

Collection: Collect seeds when ripe

Found: Cultivated

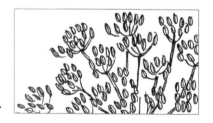

Growing: It is very easy to grow from seed.

In my area, the growing season isn't long enough to harvest the seeds, but the plant grows well for the use of leaves and bulbs for culinary use.

Action: Carminative, Anti-spasmodic, Stimulant, Expectorant

Body: Culinary, Digestive, Tonic, Nursing, Skin

Use: Food (it's one of the best herbs for digestive issues): helps dispel gas and relieves colic in babies.

Experience: People are so glad to find out that this common culinary spice has such healing powers for the digestive system because they love the unique flavor of fennel and chances are that they dislike the taste of peppermint. I have found that there are peppermint people and there are fennel people. But there are very few people who like both fennel and peppermint equally. My Italian friends were served shredded fennel bulb after large meals to help digest their food. Fennel, anise, and dill seeds all have a great ability to help the digestive system do its job. Very helpful for colicky children. Fennel seed help nursing mothers produce milk. I combine it with comfrey root to make an eye wash that works to alleviate eye infections.

Preparation: Food, Infusion, Decoction, Eye Wash

Garlic *Allium sativum*

Part Used: Bulb

Found: Cultivated

Collection: Dig when leaves die back which is mid-summer in our area.

Growing: Plant cloves in the fall for summer harvest. Pick the scapes off of greens leaves during the summer. After the leaves die back, dig up the bulbs and dry.

Action: Antimicrobial, Diaphoretic, Tonic

Body: Culinary, Immune, Circulatory

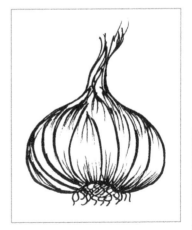

Use: Garlic is used in all cultures for culinary and medicinal use. Its anti-microbial properties are utilized by ingesting the raw cloves as well as using it in cooking. A great preventative herb, it is so healthful that there is a special preparation on the market that eliminates the smell. Garlic is good for the heart.

Experience: When nothing gets the job done, garlic is the herb to turn to. One winter, I was surrounded by all of these young adults at work and at home who kept passing a cold between themselves. Finally I had enough and insisted that they all take a spoonful of Honey Garlic Infusion every day until they got better (which they did in record time). They had had enough of being sick as well. The garlic honey mixture worked like a charm, but I have learned that a cracker or bread helps make it more tolerable for the stomach. I always keep a jar in my fridge during winter season.

Preparation: Food, Raw Garlic, Honey Infusion

Ginger *Zingiber officinale*

Part Used: Root

Collection: Grocery stores

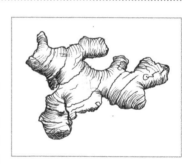

Found: Indigenous to Asia but grown throughout the world. There is an American ginger plant, *Asarum canadense,* which grows wild in the Northeast. It grows in large stands, spreading by root system. It has a beautiful flower and smells similar to Asian ginger but is much stronger. There is little information about its medicinal uses: it is a different plant altogether. It cannot be used interchangeably with the Asian ginger, *Zingiber officinale.*

Action: Anti-bacterial, Anti-viral, Anti-fungal, Stimulant, Anti-inflammatory, Diaphoretic, Anti-spasmodic, Carminative, Anti-tussive, Anti-nausea, Reproductive Tonic

Body: Digestive, Immune

Use: In food as a culinary spice which contains antimicrobial action activity against food pathogens. It treats colds and the flu, sore throats and respiratory issues. It works for digestive issues, nausea, seasickness, morning sickness, and menstrual cramps. According to Steven Buhner's book *Herbal Antibiotics*, ginger also works as an anti-tussive (calms coughing).

Experience: I use mostly fresh ginger root preparations. Fresh ginger root can be purchased in most supermarkets nowadays. I use it as a culinary spice to enhance the flavor and digestibility of food. The fresh root makes a great-tasting syrup that can be added to seltzer water to make "ginger ale". This homemade "ginger ale" is very popular for all types of digestive issues along with giving the body a "lift" which is helpful when recovering from an illness. I developed the ginger syrup recipe for people who had diet soda addictions; substituting the herbal ginger ale for their diet soda gave them the stimulating effect and sweetness of soda but was considerably healthier. It combines well with other herbs to enhance their activity. Ginger has a reputation for settling the stomach. It is very helpful for nausea. People love this herb not just because of its flavor but the complete package of how they feel when they use it.

Preparation: Food, Juice, Decoction, Syrup, Bath, Poultice

Goldenrod *Solidago canadensis* **and other species**

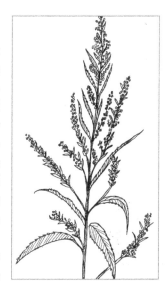

Part Used: leaves and flowers

Collection: Collect the top part of the plant just before it blooms—late summer to fall. There are many species, but you can identify the medicinal species *Solidago canadensis* by the ball-shaped "gall" on its stem during the fall. It is made by the larvae of an overwintering fly (*Eurosta solidaginis*). A friend grew up calling goldenrod the "head knocker" plant because of the ball-shaped dried stems which resemble, well, you can guess the rest. Those stems work well on people who aren't paying attention on my herb walks.

Many of the Golden Rod species flower at the same time as the ragweed plant, so many people with seasonal fall allergies think they are allergic to goldenrod when they are actually allergic to Ragweed. This green flowering plant grows in the same areas as goldenrod. It is important to learn how to identify ragweed and eliminate it from your yard if you suffer from fall allergies. I do not suggest that people *can't* be allergic to goldenrod, but it has received a bad reputation as it is probably the only plant people can identify in the fall season.

Found: Wild, Fields, Roadsides, Rarely cultivated in the Northeast

Actions: Diuretic, Antimicrobial, Anti-catarrh, Anti-inflammatory, Carminative

Body: Respiratory, Urinary Tonic

Use: Urinary and bladder issues. Can be soothing for respiratory imbalances and coughs. Used for flu and colds.

Experience: Because this plant is so common in my area, people rarely think about using it as an herbal medicine. We value something that is rare and expensive: it is human nature to believe that anything that is so common can't be any good. This plant enjoys an herbal medicinal reputation in Europe where it is not a common plant. They use Golden Rod as a respiratory and urinary tonic.

Preparation: Infusion, Tincture

Goldenseal *Hydrastis canadensis*

Part Used: Root and leaves

Collection: Endangered in the U.S. Do not pick. Buy from sustainable sources.

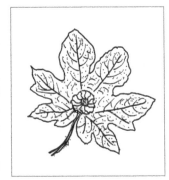

Found: Shady woodland. It is indigenous to the Northeast of the country. Growing: Can be successfully cultivated in shady gardens, woodlands or under trees. Its original habitat is Northeastern hardwood forests. It is better to start the plant from roots which can be purchased from garden catalogs. Harvest the three-year-old roots and use leaves anytime. Because the root is very expensive I have seen goldenseal leaf available for purchase. I have seen this plant cultivated successfully in a variety of habitats. There is extensive information on how to cultivate goldenseal: it is worth growing as it is one of the most expensive herbs on the market and we live in its natural habitat. Detailed growing information can be found in the book *Growing and Marketing Ginseng, Goldenseal and Other Woodland Medicinals* by Jeanine Davis and W. Scott Persons.

Actions: Tonic, Bitter, Antimicrobial, Astringent, Expectorant, Anti-inflammatory, Mucosal Tonic (helps mucous membrane disorders)

Use: Specific for the mucous membranes of body: sinuses, mouth, throat, digestive tract, lungs, and eyes. Antiseptic, it fights infections topically as well as internally. If price is any indication, goldenseal is a very sought-after herb. It has an extensive history of use by our indigenous populations. It is often teamed up with Echinacea Root in commercial preparations but I think it works in a very different manner.

Experience: This is an exceptional plant which is very popular because when used properly it works well. It works to eradicate infections that affect the mucous membranes of the body. The taste of goldenseal root is extremely bitter as a friend found out the hard way: she attempted to drink her thermos full of goldenseal infusion that she had brought to work. The best preparation to avoid the taste is to use the powder in capsules. It is the main ingredient in my recipes for cold capsules and yellow pills. I like to use it right in the beginning of a sinus imbalance. I am prone to sinus problems so I have used this plant often. It is my go-to plant for all types of sinus and throat problems. It is also used in an eyewash solution for eye infections.

Preparation: Tincture, Capsule, Poultice

Honey *Apis mellifera (honeybee)*

Part Used: Plant nectars gathered by the honeybee and stored in hives.

Collection: Local honey

Found: Local beekeepers; do not purchase honey without knowing its source.

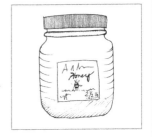

Action: Food, Tonic, Antiseptic, Emollient, Expectorant, Preservative, Skin Tonic, Burns

Use: Honey is a miracle substance. It contains the substances of local wild plants, many of which are medicinal. The bees visit these plants, gather the pollen and turn it into a substance called honey. That is why ingesting a small amount of honey every day is considered to be a type of protection for seasonal allergies. The honey introduces a minute fraction of the plant substances to the body which helps the body build up immunities to the plants that are causing the allergic symptoms. Honey contains all kinds of different substances such as protein, minerals and vitamins.

Externally it is used for all types of skin conditions. It is used internally for cough medicines, and as a sweetener for herbal preparations such as syrups. It is a very effective menstrum or liquid solvent for the honey garlic infusion I make during the cold and flu season.

Experience: In the early 90s, my college nutritional class taught me that honey was no different than sugar, a simple carbohydrate. That was actually a question on the Nutritional Board National test. (They also taught that fake fat was safe. You don't hear about that anymore.) Honey is so much more than a simple carbohydrate: it contains all kinds of substances that heal the body externally as well as internally. I use quarts of local honey for me and my grandchildren and everyone else's herbal preparations. My little granddaughter has a teaspoon of honey each day. She has always asks for a teaspoon each day like taking vitamins.

I feel it is a good preventative. I seek out local raw honey in my area and use it on a daily basis. I use it in syrups and to sweeten herb infusions and decoctions. My favorite herbal preparation is Elderberry syrup made with honey (because it tastes so good everyone takes their medicine). As I mentioned above and in the **Preventative** section, I make honey herbal infusions, the garlic infusion being my go-to honey preparation in the winter.

Preparation: Infusion, Use in infusions, Decoctions, Syrups, Skin recipes

Horehound or White Horehound *Marrubium vulgare*

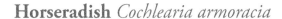

Part Used: Leaves

Collection: During the summer

Found: Cultivated

Growing: It grows well in the garden. I grew the plant for years in my garden.

Action: Expectorant, Bitter, Anti-spasmodic

Use: It has been used for centuries throughout Europe for respiratory illnesses. It has a bitter flavor. Horehound cough drops are a popular preparation.

Experience: Please refer to the introduction section on my experience with horehound and my son.

Preparation: Infusion, Candy

Horseradish *Cochlearia armoracia*

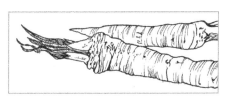

Part Used: Root

Collection: Collect the root in the fall

Found: Cultivated, Once in the garden, Horseradish can spread and become invasive.

Growing: Transplant young plants where you want them and make sure you dig all the roots up in the fall. If you leave a piece of a root in the ground in the fall it will grow into a plant the next spring (which is fine so long as you pay attention). A friend of mine didn't realize that the land he was rototilling early in the spring contained horseradish roots; subsequently, he had a garden filled with horseradish plants.

Body: Respiratory, Digestive

Action: Stimulant, Carminative, Digestive

Use: Food, Tonic, Respiratory, clears the sinuses

Experience: Horseradish is used as a stimulating food or tonic for the digestive and respiratory systems. It can clear the upper respiratory system, particularly the sinuses, more quickly than any other herb I have ever encountered. It is a good food to eat when in the recovery phase of an illness. I still remember the first time I prepared horseradish. I dug a fresh root from my garden, chopped it into small pieces and stuck it in my blender which I proceeded to put on high. I shut the blender off, removed the top and was about to take a whiff of my freshly-blended horseradish. Instead I was literally blown across the room from the powerful aroma of ground horseradish. It was so strong it took my breath away. My older farmer friends who thought that my vegetable-growing adventures were very amusing told me to cut the horseradish with white turnip if the stuff was too strong. Nowadays people are very familiar with the heat sensation of wasabi, a relative of horseradish, because of the popularity of sushi. I use horseradish in sauces. I make a large amount of a ground preparation every fall and stick it in the freezer to maintain the potency which will diminish over time. I combine horseradish root, onions, garlic, ginger root and cayenne with apple cider vinegar for a powerhouse of an herbal vinegar. See Preparation section on vinegar. It certainly keeps you warm in the winter.

Hyssop *Hyssopus officinalis*

Part Used: Leaves, flowers

Collection: Collect the upper part of the plant throughout the growing season

Found: Cultivated

Growing: Grows well in the garden. I transplant the plant by division.

Action: Expectorant, Diaphoretic, Carminative

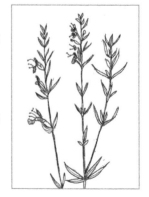

Body: Respiratory, Immune

Use: Colds, Cough

Experience: This plant, from the mint family, has a complex smell and reminds me of catnip because of its complex odor. This indicates that plant contains many volatile oils which adds to its healing properties. It combines with other respiratory herbs such as mullein for a soothing infusion for colds and coughs.

Preparation: Infusion

Lavender *Lavendula officinalis*

Part Used: Flower buds

Collections: Pick flower buds before flowers open up. This means keeping a close eye on the plants when you first see the purple bud. The buds contain more volatile oils than the ripe flowers.

Found: Gardens, cultivated

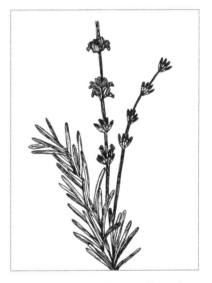

Growing: A little tricky to grow here because of our cold weather. I have had very successful lavender patches in years past. This is a Mediterranean plant so it does better in a warm dry spot; it is fussy about where it grows so if you are having trouble with your plants just move them to another spot. Sometimes that is all it takes. I add new plants every couple of years as the older plants tend to get scraggily and woody. Purchase plants at a local nursery and ask about the species that grow well in your area. I have gardening friends who grow beautiful patches of lavender here in the North Country. Their plants tend to enjoy a warmer microclimate with protection added by their proximity to a rocky fence or house.

Actions: Nervine, Carminative, Anti-spasmodic, Anti-depressive, Anti-microbial, Inhalant

Body: All over, Nervous, Digestive, Skin

Use: Used in the culinary, medical, and cosmetic worlds. The essential oil preparation is very popular. It is used topically for anxiety, depression, burns, and stress situations. Highly studied.

Experience: I use lavender essential oil in many situations. I place a drop of the diluted oil on the forehead or on the heart area for relaxation and to de-stress. This is especially effective with children. I use it in the sickroom by placing a few drops of the essential oil along with a tablespoon of water in the inhalant cup of a warm mist humidifier. The lavender essential oil is relaxing and antiseptic. I use it instead of the stronger eucalyptus essential oil which is too stimulating for use in a sick room, especially for children. I use the flower buds in a healing bath. I combine lavender with yarrow for a detoxing and relaxing bath. My favorite use is as a simple lavender oil to scent my oils, creams and salves.

Preparations: Infusion, Oil, Essential Oil, Bath

Licorice *Glycyrrhiza glabra*

Part Used: Root

Collection: Not available in North America. Purchase

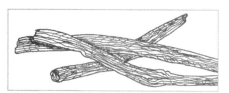

Action: Antioxidant, Relaxant, Antispasmodic, Immunostimulant, Adrenal Tonic, Anti-inflammatory, Anti-malaria, Expectorant, Demulcent, Antiviral

Body: Respiratory, Digestive, Endocrine, Skin

Use: Cold sores, coughs, lung tonic, children's recipes. The sweet taste of licorice helps masks the taste of stronger herbs in herbal preparations. I have noticed that the licorice taste isn't too strong when using it with other herbs in a recipe. It adds a demulcent and other healing actions. Many people say they do not like the taste of licorice but I would suggest you reconsider and try using it, perhaps adding a small amount to a recipe. It is used in many Chinese herbal medicinal preparations as a synergizing agent. According to the Chinese, licorice root helps the other herbs do their job. It is a much respected plant in all herbal traditions because of its multitude of actions.

Experience: Because of its antiviral properties and flavor, I use it to enhance the actions of several herbal recipes for colds and flu. I use it sparely in recipes as I do not like the taste of too much licorice. I have noticed that some people crave the taste and are so happy to enhance their recipes with licorice. A large amount of licorice root can disrupt the potassium balance in the body so it is not good for people on heart medications and other pharmaceuticals drugs. Studies suggest that it can elevate blood pressure. Occasional use of the whole herb as opposed to using stronger extract preparations is fine for most people.

The tincture preparation is unsurpassed as a cold sore preventative. Just dab a bit of licorice tincture on a beginning cold sore throughout the day; its antiviral properties prevent the sore from becoming larger. It also tastes good. I have people who never go without their supply of licorice tincture because it works so well. If you use it on herpes sores (which is the same virus), dilute the tincture with water.

Preparation: Decoction, Tincture,

Marshmallow *Althaea officinalis*

Part Used: Leaves, Flowers, Roots

Collection: Pick leaves and flowers throughout growing season, harvest roots in fall

Found: Gardens, cultivated

Growing: Grows anywhere but thrives in good soil. It loves the sandy soil of my house gardens but is not as happy with the clay soil in my big medicinal garden. Propagate by root division but it will grow from seed as well. In my opinion, it is the best all-

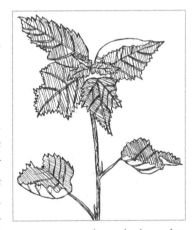

around medicinal plant to grow. If you only grow one medicinal plant this should be the plant. Marshmallow and wood betony are the plants I give away to gardeners to grow and learn to use. Find a spot for this plant in your yard. It is not fussy and looks great in a flower border with its pretty flowers.

Action: Demulcent, Expectorant, Emollient, Diarrhea, Constipation, Urinary tract infection, Cough

SECTION 4 | *Information*

Body: Tonic, Digestive, Respiratory, Skin, Urinary

Use: Root is used for soothing demulcent action on the mucous membranes throughout the body. It is the key ingredient for lung tonic and digestive tonic recipes. The leaf is used for drawing poultices for skin conditions and abscesses.

Experience: I use this plant more than any other plant in my garden. I use the roots and the leaves. The large plant is easy to harvest; the roots are plentiful. I replant some of the roots in the fall for the next season. Harvesting the leaves is easy. The leaves dry without any fuss. Sometimes I gather the leaves individually, but usually I just cut the stalks halfway through the growing season and let the leaves dry right on the stalks. By doing this, I get two cuttings in a season. The plant pops right back when trimmed. Marshmallow yields a lot of wonderful medicine for one plant. The root can be used alone or with other respiratory root herbs. It makes a soothing decoction for the mucous membranes of the body, marking it as invaluable for cough medicines, lung and digestive tonics. My favorite use for the leaves is in my sinus steam recipe. This is in my most popular herbal preparation. Marshmallow leaves are an integral part of the recipe with their soothing and antiseptic action which is released by the steam. The root was the original source of marshmallows. The root is "mucilaginous" as you will see when making a decoction. It combines with slippery elm bark and licorice as a tonic for the gastrointestinal tract.

Preparation: Infusion, Decoction, Syrup, Poultice, Steam

Mullein *Verbascum thapsus*

Part Used: Leaves, Flowers

Collection: Harvest leaves anytime but I like to gather them when the plant is young before it forms a stalk. The leaves of the new plant form a rosette on the ground. The baby plants appear in the spring and then in the fall as new plants are seeded. Collect the flowers as they appear on stalk, they ripen at different times so collect them throughout the flowering season. When you have enough, make an oil. Do not pull up the plant to harvest the flowers.

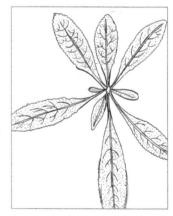

Found: Wild: fields, woods, everywhere—just look for the old stalks from the previous summer to locate new plants.

Growing: Easy to transplant to the garden if desired. They are stately-looking plants which add visual interest to a garden. Many might ask, "Why would you plant that in your garden?" I love the skeletons of the mullein plant and I leave in the garden all winter long for birds.

Action: Lung Tonic, Expectorant, Demulcent, Sedative, Vulnerary, Anti-inflammatory

Body: Respiratory, Skin

Use: The leaves were traditionally used for respiratory ailments particular for a cough, bronchitis. Externally the plants are used for skin issues like hemorrhoids and wound healing. The flower oil has traditionally been used for earaches. Native Americans smoked the leaf for cough relief. They soaked the stalks in wax and used them for torches.

Experience: I recently used mullein tea to deal with seasonal allergy cough. I had an annoying tickle of fluid dripping down which irritated the back of my throat and voice box. I needed something milder than elecampane, tastier than horehound (anything is tastier than horehound) and easy to make. Although aware of respiratory uses of mullein, I had never used it before. I was very pleased with its taste and its ease and efficiency of working. This plant is so common in our area that we overlook it which is a shame because it works so well in respiratory issues.

The traditional mullein flower earache oil is sometimes combined with the extra antimicrobial powers of garlic. Another traditional use is to shrink hemorrhoids. One of my students told me about her aunt who used mullein leaves in a steam for hemorrhoids. People used to come over to her house and she would have them sit on a bucket of steaming mullein tea for hemorrhoid relief.

Preparation: Infusion (leaves and flowers), Oil (flowers), Steam, Poultice

SECTION 4 | Information

Myrrh *Commiphora myrrha*

Part Used: Resin extract

Found: Purchase

Action: Antimicrobial, Astringent, Expectorant

Use: Colds and flu, boost white blood cells respiratory ailments, wounds, mucous membranes and skin

Experience: Cold cap recipe, taken at the first signs of illness. Combination of myrrh, oak bark, plantain tinctures for dental work.

Preparation: Tincture, Powder

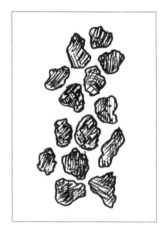

Nettles *Urtica dioica* **(Stinging nettles)**

Part Used: leaves, seeds, roots

Collection: Pick the young leaves before the plant starts to flower. Nettles emerge very early in Spring: it is traditionally picked during that season as a pot herb. The new leaves are delicious when cooked. I harvest the young leaves in the spring and the flavor of the tea is delicious. The insects love this plants and if you wait too long the leaves will be filled with holes. The leaves get increasingly tough and tough-tasting as the season

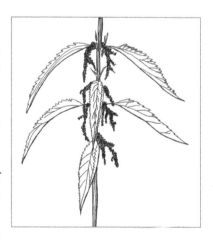

progresses. Harvest the seeds and dig the roots in fall. Nettles contains formic acid in the stems and leaves and stings when picked, hence its name: stinging nettles. Wear gloves when picking. I also wear gloves when stripping the dried leaves off the stems as well.

Found: Wild: fields. Nettles is the one plant that is commonly misidentified. People are aware of its ability to hurt so they sometimes mistake it for a thorny thistles plant or the mature prickly motherwort plant. It can be found throughout the world. It's not a plant that one forgets if you encounter it. Yellow dock leaves and plantain leaves work as antidotes to the sting. These plants are usually growing in close proximity to the nettles. Just chew up the leaves and apply to the sting.

I was on an herbal plant identification walk when a poor woman stuck her nose into the nettles patch to smell them, just as she had been doing with all the other plants. She got quite a surprise. I told her how to counteract the sting. I gave her a choice: either I or she would chew the yellow dock leaf and stick the green mass on her nose. I can't remember what she chose, going around with the sting or with a wad of chewed green plant blub on her nose.

Growing: I made the mistake of transplanting nettles to my vegetable garden. It took me years to get it out of there. Find a place where it won't spread and transplant it there. It's not fussy about its environment. It is such an important plant to have access to in the herbal world, yet the funny thing is that people hate this plant and tend to eradicate it any time they find it in their fields. My friends in the country have a new appreciation for this plant now and brew up nettle tea all winter long. It is very satisfying.

Action: Tonic, Antihistamine, Astringent, Diuretic

Use: Tonic (for the wellbeing of the whole body), Young greens in spring as nutritional food (high in protein, vitamins, and minerals). It works as an antihistamine for help with allergy symptoms. It helps remove toxins in the body so is recommended for gout and arthritis. The root is a prostate tonic; the seeds are used for male vitality. Urtification is the term for whipping arthritic parts of the body with the stinging nettles plant to bring about pain relief. No kidding.

Body: Tonic, Respiratory, Urinary, Skin

Experience: What can I say about nettles? It is so important a plant that it sounds like it is a cure-all. First of all it is a tonic: an infusion contains high amounts of vitamins and minerals. . Combined with other herbs such as oats, alfalfa, and dandelion, it's like drinking a big multivitamin pill—plus your body absorbs the tea much better than sucking down a chemical vitamin pill. Taking the time to drink a warm cup of nutritional tea brings a feeling of wellbeing in contrast to tossing back a bunch of supplement capsules.

In *Nutritional Herbology*, Mark Peterson documents the nutritional profile of dried nettles. 100 grams or one cup of dried nettles contains 2,900 mg of calcium, 860 mg magnesium, and 1,750 mg potassium along with other important vitamins and minerals.

Nettles contain antihistamines which help people with their allergies. I have heard and read that the nettles should be prepared as freeze-dried capsules in order for to enable its antihistamine effects, but I have not found this to be the case at all. A combination of ground nettles and kelp in capsule form is very helpful to combat seasonally allergies. I found that drinking a nettle infusion is also helpful, providing you are actually drinking it daily. It is important to start using nettles before the allergy season kicks in. Nettle tea is great for the elderly as it restores vigor. I once cooked up spring nettles for the family and told them it was spinach, which was a big mistake because they never trusted me again. But it was not as bad as the time I put turmeric in the macaroni and cheese (that wasn't good). Just be honest with your food preparation.

Preparation: Infusion, Powder, Tincture, Seeds

Oats *Avena sativa*

Part Used: Top part of plant: stem and spikelets or kernels. Oatmeal is made from the ripe grains contained in the spikelets.

Collection: When the plant is mature and has seeded. According to some herbalists, the optimal time for collection is when the spikelets are in the milky stage.

Found: Grown from seed. Seeds are sometimes found in small seed packages labeled Cat Grass.

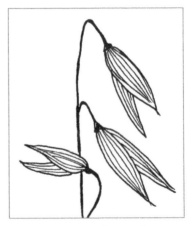

Growing: Oats are a grass and therefore very easy to grow. I broadcast or scatter the seeds in a prepared 2 x 3' plot. I then push the seeds into the soil with my boot. I put additional soil on top of the seeds and again pat it down with my boot so that it makes good contact with the soil. Then I water the seeds. In less than a week I have a hearty plot of tiny oat grass. Because you need a larger amount of seed than you do for most plants, check out local feed stores in the area for oat seeds because garden centers often only have small packages (a waste of money). I buy oat seeds in 5 lb. packages. The seed remains viable for a long time. I have used oats to ring a garden to prevent encroaching grasses which invade my vegetable gardens. In the late summer or early fall you can harvest the plants by cutting the top third, or just harvest the kernels by pulling them off the stems leaving the stems behind which can be worked into the soil. The kernels or spikelets pull off very easily and that is the desired part of the plant nowadays.

Action: Nervine, Demulcent, Soothe Digestive

Body: Tonic, Digestive, Skin, Nervous

Use: Oats are a healthy food as oatmeal or just dried oats. They make a healthy infusion which is loaded with calcium. I combine oats with nettles, alfalfa, horsetail and dandelion in my Nutritional Infusion recipe. It is my most popular infusion recipe. It contains nutrients— minerals and vita-mins—which can be taken every day. Oats are important to supporting the health of the hair and skin. Externally I use the dried plant as well as oatmeal (put into a cloth bag) in a warm bath. Oatmeal is a great vehicle to use with herb powders.

My brother had been taking a large amount of antibiotics for dental work and they were messing with his gut. He had been having diarrhea for several weeks when he called me up. I suggested that he eat oatmeal combined with two teaspoons of slippery elm powder. Both herbs would help him and his digestive tract get back in shape. I explained in detail how to make oatmeal and then how to use the herbal powder. A couple of weeks later he thanked me as he was much better. This is what he did: He took two packages of instant oatmeal, combined it with water, stuck 2-3 capsules of slippery elm powder into the oatmeal slurry and microwaved the whole thing. I was hor-rified by his preparation methods but they worked. No more diarrhea.

Experience: When I first started to use oats as an herbal plant it was called oat grass. I received a lot of ribbing when I opened up my very first 1 oz. pack-age of "oat straw" from an herbal mail order company. It smelled like it had been swept off the floor of a horse's stall. I was made fun of so much because I intended to make tea out of that little package of horse's hay—and I had actually paid real money for it. Herbal oat plants have come a long way since those days. It is possible to buy just the oat kernels or spikelets harvested at the milky stage as well as very good quality oat grass. The smell of quality oats does not resemble horse hay. It smells sweet. Oats are worth growing for the ease of growing and the nutritional benefits. I use oat spikelets and stems in my everyday nutritional teas. Every year I plant and harvest a small plot of oat grass. I eat oatmeal for breakfast. Externally I use oatmeal for baths. I grind up oatmeal into a powder and use it in herbal face and hand masks. I combine ground oatmeal with different clays and use it for skin problems.

Preparation: Food, Infusion, Tincture, Powder, Baths

Onion *Allium cepa*

Part Used: Bulb

Collection: Harvest in late summer and into fall

Found: Grow from seed or bulbs

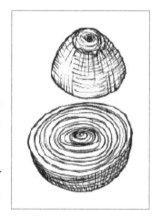

Growing: Onions are one of my favorite vegetables to grow. It is so satisfying to plant the tiny bulbs and voilà, harvest large delicious bulbs in the fall. I grow all varieties: some varieties keep in storage better than others so if you are growing a lot of onions make sure you include a variety that stores well. It seems that I am constantly chopping up an onion for some meal so I grow a lot of onions.

Action: Food, Tonic, Anti-inflammatory, Antiseptic.

Body: Tonic, Respiratory, Skin

Use: Compounds in onions enhance the nutritional content of food. Combined with honey, onions are used to make a traditional cough medicine. Onion poultices can be used on congested areas such as the chest. In *10 Essential Herbs*, Lalitha Thomas goes into detail about this versatile herbal plant.

Experience: I use onions as a tonic food anytime but especially when sick with a cold. I use onions in my Fire Cider recipe. My favorite use is in a fresh onion poultice to draw the fluid from a sprain and prevent the formation of the black and blue marks of a bruise. The drawing power of an onion is remarkable. Onions are a staple in people's kitchen so it is a great herb to study for its multitude of uses.

Preparation: Food, Infusion, Vinegar, Syrup, Poultice

Osha *Ligusticum porteri*

Part Used: Root

Found: Rocky Mountains (above 6000 ft.).

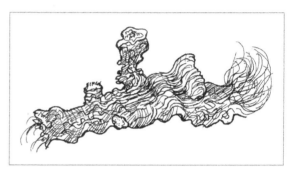

Growing: According to Richo Cech's company catalog "Strictly Medicinal Seeds", osha can be grown in many different environments; it is not limited to the high elevations of the Rocky Mountains. He sells osha seeds.

Action: Expectorant, Antihistamine, Bronchodilator, Anti-bacterial, Carminative, Diaphoretic

Body: Respiratory, Digestive

Use: Revered by Native Americans as a respiratory tonic. It is used for sinusitis, colds, allergies, and particularly throat problems.

Experience: I find that this is the best plant for throat issues. I have been using this plant in my Throat/Chest recipe for decades. I use a sparing amount of osha root in that recipe because I realized it was gathered from the wild which bothered me. Now that the seeds are available, I hope this plant will be cultivated around the country because it works so well. Its smoky taste is unique. Osha clears up the mucous in the throat; it works so well on that foggy throat feeling. It combines well with other herbs for sinus conditions.

SECTION 4 | *Information*

Combined with other strong herbs such as elecampane, it clears up long-standing respiratory infections and colds that linger after several bouts of antibiotic treatment.

Adding maple syrup as a sweetener when making a syrup helps disguise the strong taste of osha.

Preparation: Decoction, Tincture, Syrup

Passionflower *Passiflora incarnata*

Part Used: Flowers, buds, leaves, vines

Collection: When flowers are blooming.

Found: Purchase seed or plant.

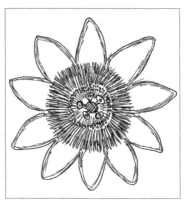

Growing: The local species *Passaflora incanata* does not do well this far north. I have tried growing it for many seasons: it is slow to appear in spring and then you never know if it will come back. One year I just gave up and stuck the roots in a pot in the fall and have had it ever since. It flourishes in a container. It grows well indoors during the cold months. It is important to bring it indoors as soon as the nights get chilly. It will continue to bloom indoors if placed in a sunny warm spot. The flowers are so unusually beautiful that it's worth just growing the plant for the beauty of the flowers. Several years ago I bought plants from a local greenhouse so I have two different species growing in pots inside; they do extremely well. I twirl the vines on a bamboo trellis so that they don't crawl up the walls (they are tenacious). In the summer, I put my plants outside. They are still flourishing after five years.

Actions: Nervine, Insomnia, Relaxant, Sedative Hypotensive, Anti-spasmodic

Body: Nervous, Circulatory

Use: Helps promote restful sleep, calm nervous conditions, and lessen pain.

Experience: I find this plant to be of benefit to most people who need a relaxant to get to sleep and stay asleep. I have taken the tincture in the middle of the night countless times to help me go back to sleep. Valerian, although very effective for sleeplessness, is not tolerated by many people, so passionflower tincture has been a blessing to many menopausal women as well as others who have trouble sleeping. I have been recommending this plant for years and by the way it flies off my shelf, I know it works. Getting a good night's sleep is the foundation of health.

Preparation: Infusion, Tincture

Peppermint *Mentha piperita*

Part Used: Leaves and Flowers

Collection: Pick leaves anytime. Pick when the plant is in bloom for the most volatile oils.

Found: Local wild species found along waterways. Many different species available in garden centers.

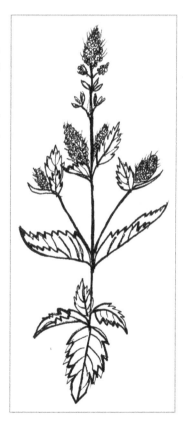

Growing: My favorite species is black stem peppermint. All species will thrive in the garden. Mint plants spread by runners so find a space that works in your garden or yard. I grow peppermint in different spots all over my yard. I am ruthless with controlling peppermint in the garden and rip up the runners every spring so it doesn't take over the garden. Some people put it in containers but I don't because the roots freeze over the winter and I don't want to buy a plant every year. Peppermint is happy to pop every spring in the garden, just give it a good pruning every year.

Action: Stimulant, Relaxant, Anti-spasmodic, Carminative, Diaphoretic, Antimicrobial, Anti-inflammatory

Body: Digestive, Respiratory, Immune, Nervous

Use: Culinary, Digestive issues: reduces nausea, calms spasms in lower intestines, stimulates the flow of bile and digestive juices, Respiratory issues, Colds and Flu, Enteric Capsules (these don't dissolve in the stomach but in the small intestines) for bowel problems. Volatile oil contains a large amount menthol. External use for irritation on skin such as poison ivy (Essential oil)

Experience: I make peppermint tincture every year. Lately I have been adding a small amount of stevia to sweeten up the taste. The combo tastes great. I use peppermint tincture or candy for cramping intestines because I am always on the go and sometimes everything cramps up. When my son was living with me, I noticed that we would go through a lot the peppermint tincture. According to my son, it works well for a hangover. Drug stores always carried peppermint oil for different uses: stomach issues, aromatics for mouth. It's important to dilute the oil because certain preparations are very strong—but then again the strong stuff is very popular.

Preparation: Infusion, Tincture, oil, candy

St. John's Wort *Hypericum perforatum*

Part Used: Flowers, leaves

Collection: Believe it or not, the flowers start to appear on St. John's Wort's Day which is June 23. I have observed this phenomenon for twenty years. Be patient and one day at the end of June you will see bright yellow flowers blooming everywhere in wild spaces throughout the area. Collect the newly-opened flowers in the morning after the dew has dried: it's best to do this on a sunny day. You will compete with the insects while collecting the flowers. The plants will reside in one area

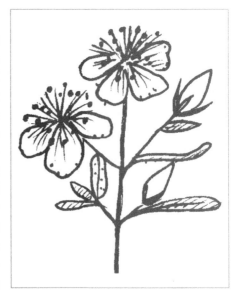

for a couple of years and then disappear. I collect the flowers throughout their flowering season which lasts about one month. See the **Preparation** section for more information on making herbal oils.

Found: Wild, fields, disturbed woodlots. Transplant plants to garden

Growing: I transplant baby plants to the garden in spring, but transferring the small plants in the fall season makes for stronger plants in the coming growing season. St. John's Wort grows well in all types of soil. The flowers and leaves contain tiny red drops of an oil soluble constituent which makes a red oil that works on the nervous endings of the skin. Your fingers will stain red as you collect the flowers. I use the buds and flowers for my oil. I use the buds, flowers and some leaves for my tinctures.

Action: Nervine, Anti-inflammatory, Antimicrobial, Anti-viral, Vulnerary

Body: Nervous, Skin, Muscular

Use: Externally, St. John's Wort works on the nervous endings of the skin and the muscles to alleviate pain. It is very effective for neuropathy. It soothes the pain of cold sores, chicken pox, shingles, and herpes sores with its antiviral action. Internally, St. John's Wort helps nervous system cope with stress and depression. It rebuilds nerve endings.

Experience: Although the oil of St. John's Wort has been made for thousand years to help calm sensitive nerve endings in the skin, the plant has become very popular in modern times mainly because of the anti-depressive action it delivers when taken internally. For the purpose of this book, I will discuss its role in alleviating pain (at which it excels). St. John's Wort oil is difficult to buy, easy to make, and boy does it work. It soothes the nerve endings of the skin as well as the nerves that are intertwined with the muscles; it helps alleviate pain such as chronic nerve pain, neuropathy, sore muscles, carpel tunnel, tennis elbow and shoulder problems. It is antiviral so it works on herpes and cold sores as well as scrapes and bruises. My favorite oil, I depend on it for so many skin issues. I love making St. John's Wort oil: the red neon color which emerges from the bright yellow flowers seems like alchemy indeed.

Preparation: Tincture, Capsules, Oil, Salve

SECTION 4 | Information

Thyme *Thymus vulgaris*

Part Used: Leaves

Collection: Collect the leaves anytime. Thyme is part of the mint family so its oils are stronger when in bloom.

Found: Cultivated, Wild species found in fields throughout the Adirondacks (look for the reddish flowers mid-Summer).

Growing: All species do well in gardens in the Northeast. I like to grow a species called "spreading thyme". It requires some maintenance because it does spread so well. I allow it to grow on the edges of my gardens. It is a sun-loving plant from the Mediterranean. I harvest the leaves all summer long. I use it fresh as soon as the leaves appear or dry for later use. It dries easily. French or English thyme grows upright as oppose to lying on the ground so it is easier to harvest (and I think a bit more potent), but I use so much thyme in my herbal recipes that the spreading thyme is better for my needs.

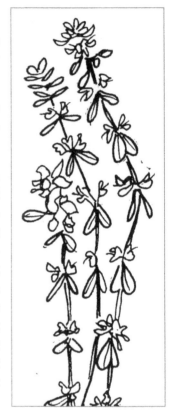

Action: Antimicrobial, Astringent, Carminative, Anti-spasmodic, Expectorant

Use: Thyme is one of the most anti-microbial and antiseptic plants. It is used in myriad ways. It is used internally as well as externally. Thyme is used in cough medicines, as well as in respiratory and digestive herbal remedies. It is an ingredient in many skin recipes because of its strong antiseptic volatile oils.

Body: Respiratory, Digestive, Skin

Experience: I use fresh thyme picked right from the garden in many culinary recipes. It adds to the flavor of dishes as well as aids with the digestibility of food. But the way I use thyme the most is as an element of my sinus steam preparation. I feel it is a key ingredient of my sinus steam. The strong volatile oils in the leaves and flowers are released into the steam and are very helpful for clearing sinus problems. It is extremely antiseptic and antimicrobial so I use the leaves in many of my cold and flu recipes. It combines well with yarrow. A note of caution on the thyme essential oil preparation: many herbal books recommend using several drops of straight thyme essential oil in a steam for the sinuses but I have received so many complaints of headaches and the drying out of sinuses that I think that the essential oil is too strong a preparation. When people switched over to using just the dry leaves for a steam, they experienced relief without any problems.

Preparation: Infusion, Tincture, Steam

Turmeric *Curcuma longa*

Part Used: Root, Rhizome

Collection: Purchase

Action: Carminative, Stimulant, Antimicrobial, Anti-spasmodic, Anti-inflammatory

Body: Muscular/Skeletal, Digestive, Skin, Liver

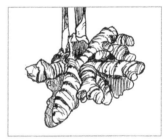

Use: Turmeric is such a versatile herb. We know it as a main ingredient of curry powder, but it is also an herbal tonic of the first degree. I recommend it to everyone: athletic types who spend time at the gym, young ladies who are runners, and to those experiencing the aches and pains of getting older. It is a tonic for the muscular/skeleton system. It is particularly effective as a bone tonic which is very helpful as we age and especially when we are involved in strenuous physical activity.

Experience: It is important to take a large enough dose of turmeric: think of it as a food. Unfortunately its taste is disagreeable to many people. I used to tell people to put the powder in their herb smoothies but for some that ruined the taste. If taste is a problem than a capsule or pill preparation will work well. Recently, I have been making Golden Milk which is turmeric paste mixed with milk, honey, nutritional oil and other spices. See the Golden Milk recipe in the Preparation section. It is a delicious way to take turmeric. It gives the body energy particularly when

SECTION 4 | *Information*

combined with other adaptagens, so it's good to take during the winter season to maintain health. Turmeric combines with other herbal roots, my favorite being ginger root.

Preparation: Infusion, Capsule, Culinary, Golden Milk

Tulsi or Holy Basil

Part Used: Leaves, Flowers

Collection: Collect the leaves and flowers during summer months into the late Fall. Collect the seeds from mature flower heads.

Found: Cultivated

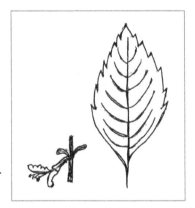

Growing: Because tulsi has become a popular daily nutritional tea around here I decided to grow it. I ordered four different types of tulsi seeds form Medicinal Plants (Horizon Herbs), an herbal seed company in Oregon. At that time the seed was hard to locate, so I bought four different types: Rama, Kapoor, Vana and Amrita. I planted the four types figuring that one type would do okay in my garden here in the North Country which is about as far away as you can get from India. That year featured an early spring and dry summer so all the plants grew well. Amrita was a burgundy color, Vana was very large and bush-like, Rama didn't do so well, but the Kapoor species thrived. It grew well all summer long, producing long stalks of purple flowers. I was still harvesting the flowers and leaves in late fall because it never stopped growing. I ended up with pounds of the dried plants. I have been growing plots of the Kapoor plant ever since. Save the flower stalks in the fall, place them in paper envelopes to dry, and harvest the tiny seeds which fall out of the stalks. I start the seeds in pots, then transfer the young plants to the garden. It grows in all types of soil but doesn't like a cold spring. Once the summer begins, tulsi thrives in my gardens.

Action: Adaptagen, Antimicrobial, Carminative, Anti-inflammatory

Use: Tulsi or Holy Basil is revered in India as a plant tonic that can be taken every day. This plant that comes from the Ayurvedic tradition works as a preventative when coming down with an illness. It helps the respiratory system do its job due to its high content of volatile oils. It is used externally for skin issues. It is considered to be a stress and anxiety reliever.

Body: Immune, Respiratory, Skin, Nervous

Experience: The tea has a spicy, complex taste that is very popular and it is an all-around tonic for the body. I serve tulsi on many occasions and people universally love the taste. I combine it with my nutritional tea blend which I drink every day. My daughter loves tulsi tea but says it makes her too mellow for her liking as she needs to be on the go during the day; I mixed her a Tulsi/ Yerba Matte herbal blend to help her de-stress but also give her an energy boost from the simulative qualities of the Yerba Matte. The combination is like an herbal Vodka Red Bull but much better for you.

Preparation: Infusion, Tincture

Valerian *Valeriana officinalis*

Part Used: Root

Collection: Collect the root in fall

Found: Fields, Gardens

Growing: Very easy to cultivate in the garden, valerian thrives in our area. It easily self-seeds all over the place once you have it in your area. The flowers have a very distinct smell in the early spring but valerian is best known for the funky smell of its dried roots. I move the baby plants that appear all over the place

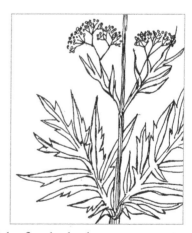

to the garden in the early spring. It is one of the first herb plants to appear in spring. The plant produces tall spring flowers which die back in summer, then the plant produces a swallow root system that should be harvested in the fall. Because you dig up the plant for its roots, it is important to plan ahead and continuously replant new plants for the year ahead.

Action: Sedative, Anti-spasmodic, Carminative

Use: One of the best sedatives in the plant kingdom. If it works for you it can be a godsend for it helps people sleep. It is specific for sleep issues. Unfortunately it does not work for everybody. For a small percent of people it can act as a stimulant. I have encountered very few people who have been affected in that way: most people that don't like valerian say that the root is too strong a sedative for their liking. It works as a strong muscle relaxant so it is very helpful when dealing with cramps, spasms and muscle-related problems. It has a history of being utilized as a strong pain reliever which makes sense.

Experience: Valerian is one of my favorite plants for relaxation and sleep. I always tell people that it got me through my son's adolescence. It really works well for me. I use both the tincture and the powder. My problem is not getting to sleep but staying asleep. I like to use capsules of the root just before bedtime: it seems to kick in during the nighttime hours when I would otherwise wake up. I have gotten out of bed in the middle of the night many times and have taken valerian tincture to fall back asleep. When I wake up in the morning I feel fine and not like I missed a night's sleep. It grows in my yard along the edges of the trees and absolutely thrives in a clay soil garden. Although harvesting the roots is more tricky than harvesting valerian roots from sandy soil. The spring flowers are 8 feet tall. They put on quite a show in the early spring. Sometimes I have to stake them because they are so tall. People complain about the smell of the roots but cats love the smell. I once smelled up a train car when I brought some fresh root in my suitcase to my aunt in New York City. It is rather potent but if it works for you the smell is not important. The tea tastes fine and not at all like the smell of the dried root.

Preparation: Infusion, Capsule, Tincture

Yarrow *Achillea millefolium*

Part Used: Flowers and Leaves

Collection: pick flower when blooming, leaves anytime

Found: fields and gardens, side of roads,

Growing: Grows profusely in garden. To start, transfer the wild plants (which can be found ev-

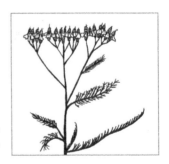

erywhere). Medicinal yarrow flowers are white in our area. If you have different colored flowers, the plants originated from a garden center and are bred for their appearance and not their medicinal qualities. It likes all kinds of soil. I use so much yarrow that I make sure I have a big patch of yarrow growing in several spots. Harvest the top part of the plant; the blossoms dry easily on the stalks. I cut the flowers all season long, and by the end of the summer I have a good supply. I have had trouble finding good quality yarrow from herbal companies so I suggest harvesting your own.

Action: Diaphoretic, Astringent, Anti-inflammatory, Anti-spasmodic, Anti-microbial, Bitter, Styptic

Body: Respiratory, Immune, Skin, Digestive

Use: According to herbalist Steven Buhner, yarrow contains over 120 constituents in this common but complex plant. In Daniel E. Moerman's *Native American Ethnobotany*, yarrow ranks in the top ten of herbal plants used by all the indigenous tribes of North America. (This book is worth reading if you are interested in learning about the ways in which native peoples used plants for just about everything.) Roman armies used this plant to heal wounds so they planted yarrow all over the Roman Empire. The astringent ability of an infusion will heal all types of skin problems. The antimicrobial and diaphoretic attributes make it valuable when dealing colds and the flu. It works as a styptic, which means that when placed on a bleeding wound it stops the flow of blood.

Experience: I use yarrow probably more than any other herbal plant. I use it in my bath when I have a cold and especially if I have the flu. It makes a great detoxifying bath and combines well with lavender and roses to enhance the bathing experience. When I moved this far North I found yarrow baths to be invaluable to warming me during the winter. I used it for my children's illnesses both internally and externally. The tea works wonders for the flu and I include it in my Traditional Gypsy Remedy along with catnip, elder flower, and boneset. Because of its anti-inflammatory and astringent qualities it works to relieve painful skin problems such as hemorrhoids and cuts and scrapes.

My favorite yarrow story comes from the time I was a fledgling herbal student and had just been taught that yarrow stopped bleeding. I couldn't believe that a plant could stanch the flow of blood. It didn't seem possible. My husband would get nosebleeds when he traveled because of the dry air. One day, he got a nosebleed when we were standing in the yard. I told him about yarrow's ability to stop bleeding and suggested that he put some in his nose. So he stuffed a whole bunch of yarrow leaves in his nose. We laughed so hard that we doubled over; the whole thing seemed so ridiculous. When he finally stood up and took the yarrow out of his nose the bleeding had stopped. We were awestruck by how it worked so quickly and thoroughly.

Preparation: Infusion, Capsule, Tincture, Herb Bath, Steam, Oil, Salve, Poultice

Chapter 21

DEFINITIONS OF PLANT HEALING SYSTEMS

In the United States we have the Western medical system of healing called **Allopathic**, Orthodox or conventional medicine. It is the current health system in this country. Herbal Medicine, Botanical Medicine or Phytotherapy utilize plants as medicines in contrast to the traditional Western medical system that promotes the use of drugs and surgery. Botanical Medicine is not taught in traditional medical schools however, with the increased attention placed on medical marijuana that may be changing.

There are numerous botanical healing systems around the world. **TCM,** or **Traditional Chinese Medicine** has many different healing modalities within that broad label. **Ayurveda** is a system of medicine with roots in the Indian subcontinent. In North America, many Native American societies utilized plants for medicinal and spiritual purposes.

For more information on this topic read *Flower Power* by Anne McIntyre. The author lists the botanical, homeopathic, flower essence and aromatherapy information for numerous medicinal plants.

Homeopathy

Homeopathy is a system of medicine that uses plants in ways differently from herbalism or botanical medicine. Homeopathy utilizes minute traces of original plant sources in preparations in the form of pills and dilutions. It was developed by Samuel Hahnemann (1755-1843), a German physician who became so disillusioned by the "heroic" methods of healing in his time which consisted of using powerful drugs (calomel or mercury), bleeding and blistering and violent purging that he quit his practice and developed a healing system that embraced an older medical theory called "like cures like". It is believed that if a plant when ingested creates a condition or symptom in the body that mimics a condition or symptom of an illness, then uses a homeopathic preparation will help the body heal from that condition. Homeopathy uses such small amounts of a plant in its preparation that it is not measureable by conventional methods. I think of it as an energy medicine that moves the body into a state of wellness.

Homeopathy works and was a very important system of medicine at the turn of the 20th century. It is very popular in Europe. Unfortunately many of its colleges in this country were closed when the American Medical Association was formed and made it its mission to close medical colleges that did not adhere with their system of medicine. Homeopathy and botantical medicine were shoved into the background, in its place was biochemistry, pharmacology and the emphasis on surgery. Currently the FDA is trying to outlaw the system of Homeopathy. That should speak volumes about its effectiveness.

Most herbalists use some homeopathic remedies. For years I have recommended a Calendula Gel that is manufactured by a US homeopathic company that was founded in 1853. This gel is very effective for skin rashes. Homeopathic teething tablets are another remedy that is extremely effective and has had decades of successful use.

Flower Essences

Flower Essences is a healing system that utilizes a homeopathic method of extracting the energy imprint of a flower – the healing vibration. In the 1930's, Edward Bach, an English doctor and homeopathic practitioner developed this system of healing using flowers. Bach believed illness was linked to stressful emotions – an imbalance between the body and the soul. His flower essences treated people's emotions as opposed to the regular homeopathic system that treated physical body symptoms. His books: ***Heal Thyself*** and ***The Twelve Healers and Other Remedies*** became the cornerstone of the flower essence healing system. His **"Rescue Remedy"** is an extremely popular essence. It is very effective in extremely traumatic situations.

The Bach system uses flowers from England. I have used flower essences that come from the North America continent. Perelandra Flower essences come from Virginia (perelandra-ltd.com), Alaska Flower essences is situated in Alaska (alaskanessences.com) and close to my home is Woodland Essence (woodlandessence.com) which is located in the Adirondack Park. Many people make their own flower essences which is a very satisfying and easy thing to do, especially if you have a special relationship to a favorite flower or plant.

Aromatherapy

Aromatherapy was rediscovered in the 1930's by a French chemist, Rene-Maurice Gattefosse, who owned a family perfume business. According to the National Association for Holistic Aromatherapy, Aromatherapy is the "art and science of utilizing naturally extracted aromatic essences from plants to balance, harmonize and promote the health of body, mind and spirit."

Using essential oils is a relatively new form of medicine that has become extremely popular. Through a steam distillation process, volatile oils are extracted from plants. These volatile oils are then diluted in a stable oil such as olive or almond oils. For instance to make an an ounce of rose oil it takes approximately sixty thousand rose petals. As you can surmised this is a very strong plant preparation and to be used with caution. Essential oils are used in baths, massage and most importantly, through the olfactory system.

The proprietors of **Adirondack Aromatherapy** in Glens Falls, NY answer questions and clear up misunderstandings regarding essential oil preparations all the time. Gretchen Morganstern, a certified practitioner of intuitive and spiritual aromatherapy through the Gritman Institute, has over 20 years' experience in working with essential oils. She stresses that ingestion can be dangerous, especially in the current culture and climate of essential oils. If taken incorrectly, some essential oils can be toxic.

For example, **Oregano Oil** has become popular for its ability to help the body fight off colds and flu. There are three different preparations that could be considered oregano oil:

- The **herbal version** is prepared by soaking the plant in oil for a period of time.

- The **supplement version** uses oregano essential oils that have been mixed with a carrier oil. This is readily available. The supplement versions are made by different companies using proprietary preparations methods. This is very confusing to the consumer because it is impossible to compare one supplement to another. Read labels to see if there are other herbs added to the oregano supplement beside the oregano plant species. In many cases the supplements contain many different plants besides the oregano herb. Check out the Latin name: Origanum vulgare on the bottles to insure that you have the correct plant. Call the company to get more information on their manufacturing processes.

🐾 **Essential Oil of Oregano** is *dangerous to take internally* because of its strength.

It is crucial to know what preparation is being ingested. Remember – it is dangerous (and in some cases, illegal) to use essential oils internally, but people do it all the time. It is especially ill-advised to give children essential oil preparations that are ingested.

COMMON NAME: LATIN NAME

Ashwagandha: *Withania somnifera*

Anise: *Pimpinella anisum*

Arnica: *Arnica montana*

Astragalus: *Astragalus membranaceous*

Boneset: *Eupatorium perfoliatum*

Burdock: *Arcticum lappa*

Black Tea: *Camellia sinensis*

Calendula: *Calendula officinalis*

Californian Poppy: *Eschscholzia californica*

Catnip: *Nepeta cataria*

Cayenne: *Capsicum frutescens*

Chaga: *Inonotus obliquus*

Chickweed: *Stellaria media*

Chamomile: *Anthemis noblis*

Cinnamon: *Cinnamomum verum*

Coffee: *Coffea*

Coltsfoot: *Tussilago farfara*

Comfrey: *Symphytum officinalis*

Cramp Bark: *Viburnum opulus*

Dandelion: *Taraxacum officinalis*

Dill: *Anethum graveolens*

Echinacea: *Echinacea purpurea* or *E. angustifolia*

Elder: *Sambucus canadensis*

Elecampane: *Inula helenium*

Fennel: *Foeniculum vulgare*

Feverfew: *Tanacetum parthenium*

Garlic: *Allium sativum*

Ginseng: *Panax quinquefolium*

Ginger: *Zingiber officinale*

Green Tea: *Camellia sinensis*

Golden Rod: *Solidago*

Goldenseal: *Hydrastis canadensis*

Hibiscus: *Hibiscus rosa-sinensis*
Horehound: *Marrubium vulgare*
Horseradish: *Cochlearia armoracia*
Horsetail: *Equisetum*
Hyssop: *Gratiola officinalis*
Kava Kava: *Piper methysticum*
Lavender: *Lavandula officinalis*
Lemon Balm: *Melissa officinalis*
Lemon Grass: *Cymbopogon flexuosus*
Lemon Verbena: *Aloysia citrodora*
Licorice: *Glycyrhiza glabra*
Marshmallow: *Althea officinalis*
Meadowsweet: *Filipendula ulmaria*
Milk Thistle: *Silybum marianum*
Motherwort: *Leonorus cardiaca*
Mullein: *Verbascum thapsus*
Myrrh: *Commiphora myrrha*
Nettle: *Urtica dioica*
Oats: *Avena sativa*
Onion: *Allium cepa*
Oregon Grape Root: *Berberis*
Osha: *Ligusticum porteri*
Passion Flower: *Passiflora incarnata*
Pau D'arco: *Tabebuia*
Peppermint: *Mentha piperita*
Plantain: *Plantago lanceolata*

Psyllium: *Plantago psyllium*
Reishi: *Ganoderma lucidum*
Red Clover Flower: *Trifolium pratense*
Red Raspberry: *Rubus idaeus*
Rhodiola: *Rhodiola rosea*
Rosemary: *Rosmarinus officinalis*
Sage: *Salvia apiana*
Schizandra: *Schisandra chinensis*
Siberian Ginseng: *Eleutherococcus senticosus*
Skullcap: *Scutellaria laterflora*
Slippery Elm: *Ulmus rubra*
Spirilina: *Arthrospira platensis*
St. John's wort: *Hypericum perforatum*
Thyme: *Thymus vulgaris*
Tulsi: *Ocimum sanctum*
Turmeric: *Curcuma longa*
Valerian: *Valeriana officinalis*
White Oak Bark: *Quercus alba*
White Willow: *Salix alba*
Wild Cherry Bark: *Prunus serotina*
Witch Hazel: *Hamamelis virginiana*
Wood Betony: *Stachys officinalis*
Yarrow: *Achilles millefolium*
Yellow Dock: *Rumex crispus*
Yerba Matte: *Ilex paraguariensis*

RESOURCES

Herbalists who write books

Bennett, Robin Rose, *The Gift of Healing Herbs*

Buhner, Stephen Harrod, *Sacred Plant Medicine, Healing Lyme*

Cech, Richo, *Making Plant Medicine*

Christopher, John, *School of Natural Healing*

Crawford, Amamda McQuade, *Herbal Remedies for Women*

de Bairacli Levy, Juliette, *The Complete Herbal Handbook for Farm and Stable*

Falconi, Dina, *Foraging & Feasting, A Field Guide and Wild Food Cookbook*

Fallon-Morrell, Sally, *Nourishing Broths*

Fallon, Sally, *Nourishing Traditions*

Gladstar, Rosemary, *The Family Herbal*

Grieve, Maude, *Modern Herbal, New York: Dover Publications*

Hobbs, Christopher, *Herbal Remedies for Dummies*

Hoffmann, David, *The New Holistic Herbal, Elder Herbal*

Howell, Patricia, *Medicinal Plants of the Southern Appalachians*

Katz, Sandor Elix, *Wild Fermenting, The Flavors, Nutrition, and Craft of Live-Culture Foods*

SECTION 4 | Information

McIntyre, Anne, *Flower Power*

Moore, Michael, *Medicinal Plants of the Desert and Canyon West: A Guide to Identifying, Preparing, and Using Traditional Medicinal Plants Found in the Deserts and Canyons of the West and Southwest*

Petersen, Mark, *Nutritional Herbology*

Puotinen, C.J., *Encyclopedia of Natural Pet Care*

Soule, Deb, *Healing Herbs for Women: A Guide to Natural Remedies*

Stamets, Paul, *Growing Gourmet and Medicinal Mushrooms*

Theiss, Peter and Barbara, *The Family Herbal,*

Thomas, Lalitha, *10 Essential Herbs*

Weed,Susun *Healing Wise*

Wood, Matthew, *The Book of Herbal Wisdom, The Earthwise Herbal*

Herbs, Herbal Products, Fungi, Herbal Plants, Seeds

Adirondack Aromatherapy
Shirt Factory, 71 Lawrence St. Glens Falls, NY 12801
www.adkaromatherapy.com
Aromatherapy Products

Adirondack Herbals
Shirt Factory, 71 Lawrence St. Glens Falls, NY 12801
www.adirondackherbals.net
Books and Herbal Products

Avena Botanicals
219 Mill Street
Rockport, ME 04856
www.avenabotanicals.com
Farm Fresh Herbs and Herbal Products

Dragon Salt Works
Shirt Factory, 71 Lawrence St. Glens Falls, NY 12801
www.dragonsaltworks.com
Himalayan Salt Products

Fungi Perfecti
P.O.Box 7634 Olympia, WA 98507
www.fungi.com
Fungi and Fungi Products

Johnny's Selected Seeds
Foss Hill Rd, Albion, ME 04910-9731
www.johnnyseeds.com
Seeds

Healing Spirits Herb, Apothecary & Education Center
9198 St. Rt. 415 Avoca, NY
www.healingspiritsherbfarm.com
Farm Fresh herbs and fungi products

Herbalist and Alchemist
51 S. Wandling Ave. Washington, NJ 07882
www.herbalist-alchemist.com
Herbal Tinctures

Jean's Greens Herbal Tea Works
225 River Street, Troy, NY 12180
www.jeansgreens.com
Herbal Products

TurtleTree Biodynamic Seed Initiative
10 White Birch Rd., Copake, NY 12516
www.turtletreeseed.org

Medicinal Plants (formerly Horizon Herbs)
Williams, Oregon
www. strictlymedicinalseeds.com
Herbal Plants and Seeds

Richters Herb Store and Nursery
357 Hwy 47, Goodwood, ON, Canada
www.richters.com
Herbal Plants and Seeds

Zack Woods Herb Farm
Hyde Park, VT
www.zackwoodsherbs.com
Farm fresh Herbs and Plants.

Woodland Essence
Adirondack Park, NY
www.woodlandessence.com
Herbal Products and Flower Essences

Flower Essences Companies

Alaska Flower Essences
www. alaskanessences.com

Bach Original Flower Remedies
Nelsons
21 High Street, Suite 302
North Andover, MA 01845
www.bachremedies.com

Perelandra Flower Essences
Jeffersonton, Virginia
www. perelandra-ltd.com

Woodland Essence
Adirondack Park, New York
www.woodlandessence.com

Websites

....

American Botanical Council: www.herbalgram.org

Christopher Hobbs, herbalist: www.christopherhobbs.com

David Hoffmann, herbalist: www.healthy.net

FDA Drug information: www.nlm.nih.govv/medlineplus/druginformation

Federal Drug Agency: www.fda.gov

Henriette's Herbal Information: www.henriettes-herb.com

Ironbound Island: www.ironbound.com

Maine Coast Sea Vegetables: www.seaveg.com

Michael Moore, herbalist: www.swsbm.com

Mrs. Maude Grieve, herbalist: www.botanical.com

National Institute of Health: www.nih.gov

Natural Products Association website: www.npainfo.org

Northeast Herbal Organization: www.northeastherbal.org

Northeast Organic Farming Association of New York: www.nofany.org

Paul Bergner, herbalist: www.medherb

The Price-Pottenger Nutritional Foundation: www.ppfn.org

United States Department of Agriculture: www.usda.gov

Weston Price Foundation: www.westonaprice.org

INDEX

NOTE: Illustrations are indicated with *italics*.
Recipes are indicated with **bold** type.

A

B

C

Drum, Ryan, 248
Dry Cough Remedy, 90, 128, **146**

dry coughs, 89–91, 128
dry heat, 66, 74

duck, 253

E

F

fruit juices, 44, 79, 80, 184, 246, 256
fungi, 56, 68, 117, 121, 252. *See also* anti-fungal herbs; kombucha beverage; mushrooms

Fungi Perfecti, 121, 252

G

H

337

I

J

K

L

labels and labeling, 160, 166–68, *167*, 263–64
lactobacillus, 218
lacto-fermented foods, 218, 250, 255
lamb, 253
larynx, 74
Latin names, 263
lavender *(Lavendula officinalis)*
...as anti-depressive, 293–94
...as antimicrobial, 293–94
...as anti-spasmodic, 293
...for anxiety, 111, 126, 294
...as carminative, 293–94
...for cold sores and shingles, 73
...for herbal bathing, 65, 229, 294, 313
...in herbal liquor, 198
...in hot packs (caution), 235
...as inhalant, 293–94
...in Materia Medica, 293–94
...as nervine, 293–94
...as scent, 294
...as sedative, 61, 104, 111
...for stress, 294
lavender essential oil, 64, 66, 67–68, 71, 88, 108, 109, 294
Laxarev, N. V., 118
laxatives, 60
leeks, 254
legumes, 253
Lemonade, 138, **150**
lemon balm
...for anxiety/calming/sleeping, 111, 112, 125, 126
...for cold sores, 72, 73, 126, 127
...as flavoring, 44

...as sedative, 104, 111, 112
...for shingles, 73
lemon drink for sore throat, 76
Lemon/Honey Remedy, 76
lentils, 253
lettuces, 254
Levy, Juliette de Bairacli, xiv
licorice *(Glycyrrhiza glabra)*
...as anti-inflammatory, 57, 106, 294
...as antimicrobial, 51, 63, 72, 86
...for children, 127, 294
...as demulcent, 42, 53, 64, 83, 284, 294
...for the digestive system, 94, 96, 296
...for dry cough, 90, 128
...for ear imbalances, 80, 130
...as expectorant, 54
...for eye imbalances, 82, 131
...as flavoring, 44
...for flu in adults, 132
...as immunostimulant, 59, 294
...as laxative herb, 60
...for lungs, 86, 87
...in Materia Medica, 294–95
...for post nasal drip, 78
...as pulmonary herb, 61, 83
...for recovery, 42, 114
...as relaxant, 294
...for runny nose, 72
...for sinus imbalance, 68, 69
...for sore throat, 76, 77
...for throat congestion, 75, 139
Licorice Tincture, 21, 72, 73, 77, 127, 138, 232, 295

liver
...acetaminophen (Tylenol) and, 34
...bitters and, 94
...dietary supplements and, 264
...formulas for, 45
...herbs for, 42, 94
...milk thistle and, 186
...pyrrolizidine alkaloids and, 85
Liver Tonic Powder, 114, 130, 137, 140, **150**
Lloyd Library and Museum, 196
local plants, 2–3
lomatium, 54
lower respiratory system. *See* lungs
lungs, 83–91
...calming coughs, 91
...clearing mucous from, 54
...congested coughs, 87–88
...congestion in, 34
...dry coughs, 89–91
...expectorants, 85–87
...function of, 63, 83–84
...herbs specific to, 83
...inhalants for, 58
...licorice for, 294
...marshmallow for, 296
...mullein for, 297
...pulmonaries and pectorals for, 61, 83
...soothing of, 50, 53, 103
...woodstoves and, 66
Lyme disease, 267
lymphatic system, 117

M

mackerel, 253, 255
macrobiotic diet, 270
magnesium, 300
Ma Huang, 265
Maine Coast Sea Vegetables, 248
Manuka honey, 190
maple syrup, 44, 100, 174, 217, 304
marigold, 275
marijuana plant (cannabis), 9–10, 101–2, 257, 261, 315
Marinol, 9–10

marjoram, 194
marshmallow *(Althaea officinalis)*, *84*
...as antimicrobial, 51
...for children's coughs, 127
...as comfrey substitute, 85, 280
...for congested coughs, 127
...for constipation, 295
...for cramping, 129
...as demulcent, 5, 11, 53, 64, 83, 85, 91, 284, 295
...for diarrhea, 129, 295

...for the digestive system, 94, 96, 99, 295–96
...for dry coughs, 128
...for ear imbalances, 80, 130
...as emollient, 295
...as expectorant, 295
...for eye imbalances, 82, 131
...for flu in adults, 132
...growing, 295
...for herbal bathing, 65
...as inhalant, 58

339

N

O

P

Q

R

Relaxation Blend, 126, 138, **151**
Relax Bath, **142**
...for anxiety/calming/sleeping, 112, 126
...for headaches, 108, 133
...for pain, 110, 135
...for recovery, 114, 137
...for sleeping, 138
Rescue Remedy, 316
resins, 51, 63, 64, 68
respiration, 63, 83–84
Respiratory Clearing Remedy, 90
respiratory system, 63–91. *See also* colds and flu; earaches and ear infections; eye infections and imbalances; lungs; mouth; nose; post nasal drip; sinuses; throat
...action of herbs for, 63–64
...allergies and, 33–34
...expectorants for congestion in, 54
...external therapies for, 65–66
...herbs for flu symptoms and, 50
...lower respiratory system, 63, 83–91
...soothing of, 5, 103
...strengthening, 61
...upper respiratory system, 63, 68–83
...volatile oils for, 306, 311
...winter season, things to watch out for, 66–68
rhodiola, 56, 120–21, 122
rhubarb, 60
rice, 235, 253
rice syrup, 44
river rocks, flat, 161, 178, *178, 179,* 180
roots, 172–74, 178, *179,* 180

root vegetables, 254
rosemary, *35*
...as antimicrobial, 51
...for congested coughs, 88, 128
...in Four Thieves Vinegar, 194
...in herbal liquor, 198
...as inhalant, 58, 65
...leaves of, 195
...for nose/runny nose, 134
...for sinus imbalance, 68, 70, 137
...in Sinus Steam, 224
...as stimulant, 62
rosemary essential oil, 64, 66, 67–68, 71, 88
roses, 65, 104, 111, 126, 229, 313
runny nose, 55, 68, 71–72, 134
rye, 253

S

safflower oil, 254
sage, *74*
...as anti-catarrh, 55
...as astringent, 64
...as carminative, 58
...in Four Thieves Vinegar, 194
...gargling with, 50, 65, 75, 77, 138, 139, 231
...as inhalant, 58, 65
...for post nasal drip, 77, 135
...in Sinus Steam, 224
...for sore throat, 12, 20, 50, 75, 76, 77, 138, 231
...for throat congestion, 74, 75, 139
sage tea, 20, 50
salad dressing, 191
salmon, 253, 255
salt
...in electrolytes replacement drink, 100
...fermented foods and, 217, 218–19, 250–51
...gargling with, 20
...in heating pads, 21, 79, 234
...in nasal wash or spray, 65, 231
...natural, 249–50, 255
Saranac Lake, New York school district, 242

Saratoga Springs, New York, 19
sardines, 255
sauerkraut, 218–21, 250, 251, 255
sauna baths, 52
scales, 160
Schizandra berry, 122
Schroon Lake, New York school district, 242
scissors, 159
sea coral, 259
sea salt, 255
seasickness, 287
seasons, eating according to, 243, 245, 254
sea vegetables, 254
seaweeds, 183, 184, 248, 249
sedative herbs. *See also* calming herbs; nervines
...catnip, 61, 104, 111, 112, 276–77
...lavender, 61, 104, 111
...lemon balm, 104, 111, 112
...marijuana, 102
...mullein, 296–97
...oats, 104, 111, 112
...passionflower, 61, 104, 111, 112, 304–5
...skullcap, 61, 104, 111, 112
...valerian, 61, 103, 104, 111, 112, 311–12

...wood betony, 104, 111, 112
seeds, 60, 253, 255. *See also specific seed names*
seltzer water, 256
Selve, Hans, 118
senna, 60
sesame, 253
sesame oil, 254
shelf life, 170, 174, 177, 180, 183
shingles, 72, 73, 307
shoulder pain, 307
Siberian ginseng, 42, 56, 105, 114, 119, 121, 130. *See also* ginseng plants and root
signature teas, 28–29
simple recipes, 166
Sinus Clearing Remedy, **152**
...for congested coughs, 87, 127
...for dry coughs, 90
...for ear imbalances, 80
...for headaches, 133
...for nose/runny nose, 71, 134
...for post nasal drip, 77
...for sinusitis/sinus problems, 69, 137
...for throat congestion, 74, 139
sinuses. *See also* post nasal drip
...allergies and, 33–34, 68, 222

U

V

vitamins and minerals. *See also* dietary supplements, herbs as
...good food choices for, 254
...in herbal smoothies, 186
...in honey, 290
...in nettles, 299–300
...in oats, 301
...Recommended Dietary Allowances, 257–58
...in tonic herbs, 245–46

vodka, 194, 196, 197, 202
voice box. *See* larynx
volatile oils
...antimicrobial, 51, 93
...in carminative plants, 58, 95
...in chamomile, 93
...digestive system and, 58, 93, 95
...extraction of, 317
...in hyssop, 293
...infusions and decoctions and, 157, 168
...in peppermint, 93, 305, 306
...steaming sinuses and, 70, 222
...in thyme, 308–9
...in tulsi (holy basil), 311
vomiting, 99–100, 140
vulnerary herbs, 279–80, 296–97, 306–7

W

walnuts and walnut oil, 253, 255
water, 17, 19, 37–38, 168, 198, 245, 256
water-based preparations, 13, 26
weight loss industry, 265–66
well-being, physical, 56
Weston A. Price Foundation, 240
wheat, 253
wheat grass, 254
whey, 251
white blood cells, 4, 39, 298
white horehound. *See* horehound or white horehound (*Marrubium vulgare*)
white tea, 266
wild cherry bark, 54, 64, 83, 91, 128

wildcrafting, 2
Wild Fermenting (Katz), 250–51
wild rice, 253
wild sarsaparilla, 119
willow bark, 57, 106, 108, 109, 135
wine, 197–98
Winter Root Cider, **192–94**
...for congested coughs, 128
...for eye infections, 131
...preparation of, 191–94, *193*
...as preventative/at first sign of illness, 136
...for recovery, 137
...for sore throat, 76
...as tonic, 140

winter season, things to watch out for, 66–68
wirewhisks, 159, *178,* 180
wood betony, *112*
...for anxiety/calming/sleep, 111, 112, 125, 126
...growing, 295
...for headaches, 107, 132, 133
...as relaxant, 107, 126
...as sedative, 104, 111, 112
Woodland Essence, 317
woodstoves, 66
wormwood, 194
wound healing, 190, 209, 280, 297, 298, 313

Y

yarrow (*Achillea millefolium*), 12, 52, 89
...as anti-carrarh, 55
...as anti-inflammatory, 57, 106, 313
...as antimicrobial, 11, 51, 313
...as anti-spasmodic, 313
...as astringent, 64, 313
...as bitter herb, 313
...for congested coughs, 87, 88, 128
...as diaphoretic, 46, 52, 64, 79, 229, 313
...for dry coughs, 91, 128
...for ear imbalances, 80, 130
...for flu, 132, 275, 283, 313

...growing, 312–13
...for headaches, 133
...for herbal bathing, 18, 46, 52, 65, 70, 79, 81, 229, 294, 313
...in Materia Medica, 312–14
...for nose/runny nose, 71, 134
...for prevention/first signs of illness, 60, 136
...for sinusitis/sinus problems, 70, 137
...as styptic, 313–14
...for throat congestion, 139
...thyme used with, 309
...in Traditional Gypsy Flu Remedy, 50, 313
...for whole body, 12

...for wound healing, 313
yeast, nutritional, 184, 186
yellow dock, 60, 299
Yellow Pills, **156,** 180. *See also* Cold Caps/Yellow Pills
yerba matte, 62, 105, 311
yogurt. *See also* dairy products
...as fermented food, 218, 250
...gelatin added to, 209
...as good food choice, 253, 255
...in herbal smoothies/shakes, 46–47, 177, 184–86, 246
Young's Rule, 31